e-learning for GP Educators

T0133873

Edited by

John Sandars

Senior Lecturer in Community Based Education
Medical Education Unit, School of Medicine, University of Leeds

Foreword by

Mayur Lakhani

Chairman of Council
Royal College of General Practitioners

Radcliffe Publishing
Oxford • Seattle

Radcliffe Publishing Ltd
18 Marcham Road
Abingdon
Oxon OX14 1AA
United Kingdom

www.radcliffe-oxford.com
Electronic catalogue and worldwide online ordering facility.

British Library Cataloguing in Publication Data

A catalogue record for this book is available from the British Library.

ISBN-10 1 84619 011 8
ISBN-13 978 1 84619 011 7

Typeset by Anne Joshua & Associates, Oxford
Printed and bound by TJ International Ltd, Padstow, Cornwall

Contents

Foreword

e-learning is an exciting opportunity to drive up standards of patient care by finding innovative ways of supporting GPs in their efforts to keep up to date. A high quality learning experience with an emphasis on improved patient outcomes is what we should be striving for. I am delighted to be able to write the foreword for this publication which I regard as 'leading-edge'. I am particularly pleased to see the foundations of e-learning so clearly laid out. The book covers issues such as quality assurance, standard setting, support for learners, blended learning, research and measuring effectiveness. The world of e-learning is changing and once again general practice is leading the way in devising solutions. I believe that e-learning will become even more important if the strategy outlined in this book is followed.

The Royal College of General Practitioners is the largest medical royal college in the UK. Established in 1952, it has led the way in driving up standards in general practice by promoting the education and training of GPs. Healthcare professionals are now clearly expected to demonstrate accountability for the standard of their work to patients, their peers, the health service and regulators. Integral to this is a sound system of continuing professional development.

As a GP appraiser, I know that the importance and impact of a high quality learning experience cannot be underestimated. These are, however, far and few in between! And as a practising GP I also know just how hard it can be to keep up to date in a generalist discipline and showing progress. Having access to information is the straightforward bit – processing it and embedding it into clinical practice is the much bigger challenge as this book rightly points out. Improvement is distinctly possible if GP learning is supported properly. As a user of e-learning, I know how useful this technique can be if undertaken properly and to a defined standard.

I have been interested in the issue of e-learning and so on 15 March 2005, the RCGP, working with John Sandars and others, designed and hosted the first ever primary care conference in e-learning.[1] Many of the themes of the conference are covered in this excellent book. The RCGP continues to engage with this area through its distance learning unit that provides supported multimedia distance learning for professional development.[2]

I have previously written elsewhere that professional development is a process whose potential has not been fully realised and as Chairman of the RCGP, I want to modernise the process. I have no doubt that this book will be a valuable contribution to that modernisation process to create an innovative learning culture and society in healthcare.

Dr Mayur Lakhani FRCGP
Chairman of Council
Royal College of General Practitioners
London
June 2006

Notes

1 www.medicalnewstoday.com/medicalnews.php?newsid=21203 [accessed 3 January 2006].
2 www.rcgp.org.uk/learning/index.asp.

Preface

e-learning is here to stay! It is not a passing fad that will fizzle out in the next few years. Many GP educators are sceptical of its value but there is now increasing evidence that shows that e-learning can be as effective as more traditional methods. It is now time for attention to be directed towards finding the place of e-learning in education for primary care and this is the aim of the book.

In this book you will find a collection of readings that reflect the current experience of enthusiasts who have wrestled with the challenge of introducing e-learning into a wide variety of primary care education settings. Some ventures have been highly successful – some less so! This is the reality and not the hype that often surrounds e-learning. I hope that everyone who reads this book will become a little wiser about e-learning and help other educators and learners to see its enormous potential. The world of e-learning is rapidly evolving and I have tried to provide a snapshot of current evidence and practice. I have chosen authors and topics that reflect the main approaches that are used for continuing professional development, rather than in academic institutions.

The initial chapters outline the wide range of e-learning approaches and the evidence base on how it has been used by general practitioners. An essential aspect is the learner experience and a personal perspective of e-learning is offered by an established GP. Effective e-learning requires practical application of educational theory and this is discussed, especially the importance of the social aspects of learning.

Most GP educators will be in positions where they recommend e-learning. A clear guideline on how to choose an e-learning product is provided and the complexity of the current approach to accreditation is clearly explained. This is followed by several examples of how high quality e-learning can be provided and the variety of different approaches that have been used.

Some GP educators will have more need for practical advice on how to use e-learning in their work. A series of chapters offer useful advice on how to implement e-learning that is based on the extensive experiences of the authors.

The final chapters offer an exciting glimpse into the future of e-learning and a European perspective. A final chapter provides an overview of the challenge of research in e-learning. Real world research is an essential activity to inform the development of e-learning in primary care.

Many of the chapters are based on articles that have been previously published in *Education for Primary Care* and *Work Based Learning in Primary Care*. I thank Radcliffe Medical Publishing and the respective editors, John Pitts and Jonny Burton. Both John and Jonny have also been great supporters of e-learning over the years and have devoted regular space in their already packed journals.

I would like to especially thank all of the authors and the production team at Radcliffe Publishing. It has been a real privilege to learn from the experiences of my e-learning peer group. This book would still have been a twinkle in my eye without their enormous support.

The future of e-learning in primary care does rest in your hands. You may be someone who is an educator, or a learner, but you can influence the future direction of e-learning for primary care. An overall, and major, theme is that effective e-learning requires interaction with colleagues. There is also a consistent thread that e-learning should be driven by educational principles and not the latest technology. Happy reading, and I hope that you will find a place for e-learning in your work and life.

John Sandars
Leeds
June 2006
j.e.sandars@leeds.ac.uk

About the authors

Editor

John Sandars MBChB (Hons) MSc FRCGP MRCP CertEd Diploma in Counselling Diploma in Palliative Medicine
Senior Lecturer in Community Based Education, Medical Education Unit, School of Medicine, University of Leeds, Leeds

John developed an interest in the educational potential of e-learning whilst developing a CD-ROM several years ago. This interest led him to become a member of the team that developed the first UK web-based Masters in Population Health. He was Director of the E learning for Health Unit in the Evidence for Population Health Unit at the University of Manchester, where he also developed and evaluated online learning networks for a range of healthcare professionals. He has a major interest in both practical and research approaches to e-learning. He regularly writes a column (the e-learning site) in *Education for Primary Care* and has written several articles in *Education for Primary Care*, *Work Based Learning in Primary Care* and *BMJ Careers*. His research interests are mainly about online communication and the use of new technologies to enhance learning.

Contributors

Zoe Barker is Legal Director for DoctorOnline.nhs.uk. She qualified as a city solicitor and joined Doctor Online in 1998.

David Bossano MBBS MRCGP
The Robert Darbishire Practice, Rusholme Health Centre, Manchester

David is a part-time GP and clinical lead at a large inner-city practice. He learns from and is supported by discussions with his colleagues on work email. He is a student on the online Masters degree in Population Health.

Sue Lacey Bryant BA (Hons) Dip Lib MSc, MCLIP
Doctors.net.uk, Abingdon, Oxon

Sue's contribution to the development and evaluation of the Doctors.net.uk model of e-CME is informed by an understanding of the learning needs and preferences of GP educators and registrars gained 'at the coal face' in practice. An independent health information specialist, Sue has a background in producing and evaluating multimedia learning materials and in information skills training. Sue is familiar with working in virtual learning environments and fully committed to promoting effective e-learning. An experienced peer reviewer with extensive experience of writing for the web, Sue has a practical grasp of the benefits and pitfalls of e-learning derived from her experiences as an e-tutor and an e-learner.

Jonathan Burton MA MBChB MRCGP
Editor, *Work Based Learning in Primary Care* and Associate Director, London
Deanery, London

After a degree in English Literature, Jonny qualified in medicine, did hospital
jobs and then worked in South America as a medical volunteer. He was a partner
in an Essex general practice until retirement and he now works as a part-time GP.
He has been a GP educator for 20 years and is currently Associate Director in the
London Deanery responsible for facilitating educational research and editor of
Work Based Learning in Primary Care. Jonny has co-edited two books published in
2003 – *Work Based Learning in Primary Care* and *Supervision and Support in Primary
Care*.

Rachel Davey BSc MMedSci PhD
Professor in Physical Activity for Public Health, Faculty of Health at Staffordshire
University, Stoke-on-Trent

Rachel has developed online distance learning courses and CPD for health
professionals and currently runs the Master of Public Health and MSc in Physical
Activity and Public Health Awards. These are innovative, tailored to individual
need and integrated within the workbase, have minimal face-to-face requirements and are designed so that the student can jump off – or back on the skills
escalator at any point.

Nick Foster FRCGP DCH DRCOG BDS
General Practitioner and Course Organiser, Nottingham Vocational Training
Scheme

Nick has set up and managed the scheme website www.nottm-vts.org.uk since
2000. Teaching has now developed into a paperless e-learning environment,
encouraging the use of IT and the internet as a resource tool for teaching and GP
registrar education.

He has been an examiner for MRCGP membership since 1996.

Dr med **Jochen Gensichen** MPH
Institute for General Practice, Johann Wolfgang Goethe University Hospital,
Frankfurt am Main, Germany

Jochen is a qualified General Practitioner and has a Master of Science in
Education and a Master of Public Health. He is Head of the Chronic Care and
Health Services Research Unit at the Institute of General Practice, an original
member of the Network E-Learning in General Practice (ELA), Member of the
German Society of General Practice and Family Medicine (DEGAM) and a Member
of the German Association of Medical Education. He has particular interests in e-
learning in medical education (www.e-learning-allgemeinmedizin.net), case
management for depression in primary healthcare (www.prompt-projekt.de),
chronic care in primary healthcare (www.chronic-care.de) and evidence-based
guidelines for general practice.

Alex Jamieson MA MBChB
Associate Director, London Deanery, and Course Director, MSc in Primary Care,
Queen Mary's School of Medicine and Dentistry, London

Alex has a practical as well as an academic interest in e-learning, and has
written on the subject in the past, having been co-author of a chapter on
'Information, Learning and New Technologies' in *Guide to Education and Training*

for Primary Care (Oxford University Press, 2002) and in his column on e-learning during 2003–2004 in the journal *Work Based Learning in Primary Care*.

Peter Johnson MMedEd MRCGP DCH DRCOG

Peter has been a GP in Cheshire for nearly 12 years and was GP Tutor for the Halton area for more than 10 years. He completed his MSc in Medical Education in the 2001 and subsequently became a distance learning e-tutor for Cardiff's Postgraduate Certificate in Medical Education (PCME) students. More recently he has been involved in developing the e-learning branch of the Mersey Deanery (General Practice) website and has developed e-learning courses for non-principals and hospital junior staff.

Michele Langlois BSc (Hons) MSc PhD

Michele worked as a Research Associate in the E-learning for Health Unit at the Evidence for Population Health Unit at the University of Manchester. In this unit she was part of the team that developed and evaluated the first UK web-based Masters in Population Health and online learning networks for a range of healthcare professionals. This work has led to several joint publications on e-learning. Currently, Michele is a private research consultant specialising in public health research based in the North West of England.

Jennifer McDonough RGN

Jeni trained at Guy's Hospital and was a ward sister until leaving to start a family. She returned to nursing in 1982 as a practice nurse and has recently retired after 23 years at the same practice. She has been a contributor to the journal *Work Based Learning in Primary Care*, reflecting on the changes in the education and development of practice nurses. Jeni continues an interest in practice nursing by undertaking part-time locum work.

Richard McDonough MA BSc

Originally qualified as a chartered quantity surveyor, he made a career change when he was appointed a GP fund holding manager 1996, using his transferable financial skills and management experience. Following the abolition of the NHS internal market he took on the role of practice manager. He has an AMSPAR Diploma in Practice Management and an MA in work-based studies (primary care development). Richard is currently acting chief examiner for the AMSPAR Diploma in Primary Care Management and an assistant editor for the journal *Work Based Learning in Primary Care*.

Anne McKee PhD MA PGCE BA

Assistant Editor, *Work Based Learning in Primary Care* and Head of Centre for Educational Development, Open University

Anne is an educationalist, specialising in curriculum evaluation and research in medical and health sciences education. Over a 15-year period, her research has brought her into primary care, hospital and university settings, examining how the NHS has become a different place in which to work and learn and how health professionals are taught. Both her research and writing identify the challenges and opportunities of improving practice-based professional education. Key to this is rethinking the relationship between policy, research, learning and teaching and real practice. Increasingly, she searches for new ways in which higher education can support professional learning. As Head of the Centre for Educational

Development (CED) at the Open University, she is designing courses to improve learning and teaching and utilising technologies to make these accessible. Those courses link teaching and research. Anne is deputy editor of *Work Based Learning in Primary Care*, published by Radcliffe Medical Press, and a member of the Editorial Board of *Health and Social Care*, published by Blackwell Science.

Gary Motteram BA MEd
Senior Lecturer, School of Education, University of Manchester, Manchester
   Gary has worked in traditional classrooms as well as developing distance and online materials. He is interested in providing good quality experiences in whatever context he and the learners find themselves in. His main work is training language teachers, but more recently has taken on the management of more general e-learning projects and managed the eChina UK project for HEFCE.

Maura Murphy BMed Sci, MB ChB MRCGP, DipMedEd, Certificate Primary Care Facilitation, ECDL, Certificate in e-Learning Tutoring Skills
Sessional GP and previously a Postgraduate GP Tutor, Mersey Deanery, Liverpool
   Maura contributed to the book since she thinks that e-learning is a way ahead for future learning in medicine as elsewhere. She regards it is a fascinating time-saving medium which can reach out globally, and this is why she became an e-learning champion in her area and then went on to develop tutoring skills to use online. Besides which it is good fun!

Tim Ringrose BSc (Hons) MB BCh MRCP
Doctors.net.uk, Abingdon, Oxon
   Tim is Director of Professional Relations for Doctors.net.uk. Tim joined Doctors.net.uk after training in nephrology and intensive care at Oxford. He is an Honorary Senior Lecturer at the Medical School, University of Warwick, and a member of the Centre for Evidence-Based Medicine at Oxford.

Dr med **Andreas Christian Soennichsen**
Director of the Institute of General Practice, Family Medicine and Prevention, Paracelsus University, Salzburg, Austria
   Andreas is an original member of the Network E-Learning in General Practice (ELA), Member of the German Society of General Practice and Family Medicine (DEGAM) and Member of the German Society of Clinical Nutrition. He is interested in the integration of clinical case studies in preclinical medical education and is keen to optimise patient care in general practice and to improve medical education inside and outside of the university setting.

Andrew Thornett MRCGP FRACGP FACRRM CertMedEd
General practitioner and Senior Clinical Lecturer in Medical Education, Stafford-shire University, Stafford
   Andy is a general practitioner in Tamworth, with postgraduate training and qualifications in psychiatry and child health. He trained as a GP in Nottingham-shire, before working in Southampton as a Clinical Research Fellow. He then spent a year in rural and remote South Australia before joining Staffordshire University as Senior Lecturer in Medical Education. Andrew has a particular interest in blended learning approaches in health and social care education and making the best use of learning to suit personal development needs. His roles

include e-learning development in the Faculty of Health and Sciences at Staffordshire University.

Dr med **Horst Christian Vollmar** MPH
Competence Centre for General Practice and Outpatients' Health Care Witten/ Herdecke University Witten Germany

Horst is a qualified GP and has a certification in Medical Informatics. He is an original member of the Network E-Learning in General Practice (ELA), and a member of the guideline working group of the German Society of General Practice and Family Medicine (DEGAM). He has a particular interest in e-learning for continuing medical education (www.medizinerwissen.de, www.leitlinien-wissen.de) and knowledge translation. He has conducted a randomised trial to compare a blended learning approach about dementia with a conventional training programme in primary care quality circles.

Dr med **Uta-Maria Waldmann** MRCGP
Department of General Practice, University of Ulm, Ulm, Germany

Uta-Maria is an original member of the Network E-Learning in General Practice (ELA) and a member of the German Society of General Practice and Family Medicine (DEGAM). She qualified as a general practitioner both in Great Britain and Germany. She has a teaching and research post at the University of Ulm with special interest in decision making in general practice and e-learning in medical education (www.e-learning-allgemeinmedizin.net). Her current research in- volves e-learning and e-exams: teaching and assessment with virtual patients.

Kieran Walsh MB BCH BAO DCH MRCP
Clinical editor at BMJ Learning (www.bmjlearning.com). This is the educa- tional website of the BMJ Publishing Group. He worked as a clinician for a number of years before moving into the field of medical education. He teaches communication skills for the membership of the Royal College of Physicians examination and actively participates in examination paper setting for the membership of the Royal College of Physicians of Ireland examination.

Chapter 1

What is e-learning?

John Sandars

Key points

- e-learning delivers learning by any form of electronic media.
- The main impetus has been the development of new technologies.
- m-learning, using mobile technology, is an exciting recent development in e-learning.
- There are potential benefits to both the learner and the educational provider.

Introduction

There is some debate about an exact definition of e-learning, or electronic learning, but a useful definition is 'the delivery of learning via any form of electronic media'.[1] This simple definition neatly encapsulates the two dimension of e-learning: technology and education.

The technology

There are two main reasons to start with technology. First, the development of e-learning owes itself to the exciting potential for technology to be used in education, and second, there has been dominance in the development of e-learning by technical experts.

Learning content can be offered in different formats, such as text or video images, and electronically delivered via a range of technologies. The quality of the different formats can be extremely high and often they are often combined to ensure maximum effect – so-called 'multimedia'. The benefit of the wide range of different technologies is that it offers ease of access to learning content 'any time and any place', and the opportunity to choose from a variety of formats and delivery systems. Technology can be used to not only store and deliver content but allow quick access to resources via the internet. In addition, it can provide opportunities for interaction between tutors and learners and between groups of learners.

Most e-learning relies on the learner sat at a static computer. The e-learning content can be delivered locally by the use of CD-ROMs or more widely by using the internet to access web-based resources. The internet also allows communication between individuals. This approach provides content of high visual and auditory quality. The main disadvantage is the limited opportunities for access to the static computer.

Recently, newer technologies have enabled access at literally 'any time and any place'. This has been called 'm-learning', or mobile learning.[2] Examples of mobile technology include:

- notebook (laptop) computers
- Personal Digital Assistant (PDA)
- cellular phones
- smart phones, combining a PDA and a cellular phone.

The importance of this approach is that there has been phenomenal growth in the use, and development, of mobile technology and this trend is expected to continue. This creates exciting learning opportunities. The small screens cannot deliver very high quality visual images but are very useful for taking small 'bite size' pieces of educational content, such as a revision topic, whilst waiting at a bus stop.

The education

Essentially e-learning is distance, or distributed, education. The original distance educators and learners relied on the postal system but now they rely on sophisticated technology. An important aspect of this approach to learning is that the learner has a greater degree of control of how, when and where their learning takes place. Learning resources can be accessed at a time and place convenient to the learner. This has obvious advantages but there is usually less direct contact with tutors and fellow learners compared with a course that is delivered face to face.

The rapid development of e-learning has clearly focused attention on the underlying philosophy of the educational approach, the so-called pedagogy.[3]

Behaviourist approaches

Computer-based training was one of the earliest forms of e-learning in which the learner was given a programmed sequence of tasks. This approach has become less of a feature in e-learning. The main characteristic of this approach to learning is the provision of information without any appreciable interaction with the learner.

Cognitive constructivist approaches

Building on existing knowledge is the distinguishing feature of this educational method. This approach is facilitated by active involvement of the learner in the learning process, such as tasks, self-tests and learning exercises. Most web-based and CD-ROM-based approaches make extensive use of this method, often with the help of multimedia stimuli.

Social constructivist approaches

This method recognises the importance of interaction with other learners to share and build knowledge. This can be facilitated by the use of technology that allows collaborative learning, such as email or discussion boards.

Combining technology and education

The potential for e-learning can only be achieved if an approach is used that concentrates on the education and recognises that the role of technology is to enhance the learning, rather than trying to find educational uses for new technology.

The ideal process for developing an e-learning approach is to identify the main learning outcomes that are needed, then decide on how these can be met by using the available technology, to choose an appropriate technology for the learner and the learning outcomes and finally evaluate the design and implementation process so that it can be improved.[4]

Formal and informal learning

Informal learning is self-directed by the learner and occurs outside the often rigid boundaries of institutions and professional bodies. Learners identify their own learning needs, usually by active participation in professional activities. There is an attempt to meet these learning needs by a variety of methods. Important informal methods of e-learning include participation in internet-based discussion forums and searching websites for information ('surfing').

Formal education has tended to provide specific courses, usually over a protracted period of time, but many professionals require more informal approaches when they can take small amounts of learning content at the time when it is required. This is often called 'just in time' learning.

Asynchronous and synchronous methods

Most collaborative learning online uses asynchronous communication, where messages occur over a period of time. This is typical of email and discussion boards. A useful analogy is the posting of messages on a wall and these are read, and responded to, by other group members as and when they wish. Some users find this helpful, allowing them to reflect on the messages, but there is increasing interest in methods that allow synchronous communication. In synchronous methods, communication occurs in 'real time'. Examples include the chat rooms available on many internet websites, such as MSN Messenger.

Blended approaches

The advantages of e-learning have become increasingly recognised but there are often barriers to fully implementing e-learning as an educational approach. These barriers include the need for resources, both human and financial, but also the acceptance by both tutors and learners. This has led to the concept of 'blended learning' in which e-learning approaches are used to supplement more traditional methods.

The advantages of e-learning for the educational provider

There has been great emphasis on meeting the needs of the learner (and rightly so) but e-learning can offer many advantages to the educational provider. These include:

- ease of updating course material
- ability to offer a wide range of learning approaches and topics
- less need for expensive physical resources, such as lecture theatres and libraries
- attract students for a wider area, including international
- ease of transfer of small units of course materials between courses
- opportunity to integrate e-learning with more traditional methods of course delivery, so-called 'blended learning'.

e-learning in other contexts

A recent review of e-learning in higher educational institutions in the United States noted that over 1.6 million students took at least one online course in the Autumn of 2002, 97% of public institutions offered at least one online course and 57% of academic leaders felt that learning outcomes for online education were equal or superior to face-to-face instruction.[5] In a recent article by Donald Klein and Mark Ware, it was noted that the annual growth rate for the use of e-learning for continuing professional education by various types of professionals, including lawyers, accountants, surveyors and healthcare professionals, in the United States was currently 100%.[6]

Conclusion

e-learning is a relatively young approach to education but it can offer exciting learning opportunities for learners if technology is appropriately used to enhance the learning experience. It is readily apparent that e-learning is not simply one approach. It is composed of a variety of methods which can be 'mixed and matched' depending on the requirements of both the educational provider and the learner.

The potential is already being recognised in the United States and it needs only time for e-learning to become more widely established in other countries. The future direction of e-learning for general practice will be determined by major policy initiatives in the United Kingdom. This is the result of the government's education, National Health Service (NHS) and technological agendas.[7] Changes are already starting to take shape. Each Strategic Health Authority should have developed a five-year e-learning strategy and this is a key part of the national lifelong learning strategy that was launched in 2001. It needs only time before GP educators will have to fully respond to the challenge.

References

1 Snook A (2005) On-line Learning – the Eye of the Storm. *e-learning zone* (www.e-learningzone.co.uk/feature6.htm).
2 Abernathy DJ (2001) Get ready for M-Learning. *Training & Development.* **55**: 20–22.
3 Broadbent B (2002) *ABCs of e-Learning.* Jossey-Bass/Pfeiffer, San Francisco.
4 Allen MW (2003) *Michael Allen's Guide to E-Learning.* John Wiley and Sons, Hoboken, New Jersey.
5 Allen IE and Seaman J (2003) *Sizing the Opportunity: the quality and extent of online education in the United States.* Sloan Foundation, New York.
6 Klein D and Ware M (2003) E-learning: new opportunities in continuing professional development. *Learned Publishing.* **16**(1): 34–6.
7 Sandars J (2003) e-learning: the coming of age. *Education for Primary Care.* **14** (1): 1–5.

e-learning for general practitioners: lessons from the recent literature

John Sandars and Kieran Walsh

Key points

- Most studies have been performed outside the United Kingdom and include small numbers of participants.
- Only two studies resulted in changes in clinical or professional behaviour.
- No studies compared different methods of e-learning.
- General practitioners (especially rural ones) liked e-learning, especially the sharing of experiences with other colleagues and the opportunity to work at their own pace.
- Technological problems are a barrier to implementing e-learning, with many learners having low competence and confidence in the use of information technology.

Introduction

In this chapter we describe the results of a review that we performed of the published literature of e-learning for general practitioners. Our aim was to identify the evidence base of e-learning for general practitioners so that future developments and policy decisions could be appropriately informed.

We gathered information by searching Medline (1998–2003) and Embase (1998–2003) using the MeSH terms: 'computers', 'computer communication networks' and 'electronic mail' in combination with 'education, medical' and 'education, distance'. Only articles in English were included in the search.

Only studies from 1997 were included since we regarded studies prior to this date as not being relevant to the present state of e-learning. Over the last six years there have been rapid developments in e-learning, both in the provision of content and in the use of highly sophisticated information technology.

We identified 352 articles from both databases. We read the titles and abstracts of these articles. We only included articles that were relevant to e-learning for general practitioners, either for continuing professional development or for use in training future general practitioners. We excluded those that related to undergraduate education, use of training simulators, education management systems, computer-based testing, clinical decision support systems and telemedicine without a specific education component. We also excluded all articles that described training and continuing professional development in secondary care and in other healthcare professions. We identified 45 articles that were relevant to the review.

Our findings

We found no studies that evaluated the use of personal digital assistants (PDAs). No systematic reviews were identified. All studies included general practitioners as participants, but some studies also included general practitioners in training.

The use of internet approaches

We found seven studies that evaluated internet approaches, with learning opportunities being provided by online methods.

A randomised controlled trial of an interactive case-based education programme for managing domestic violence was compared with an intensive classroom-based programme.[1] The researchers used an externally developed and validated pre-test/post-test instrument to assess learning in the 65 physicians who participated. The online programme improved physician confidence and beliefs in managing domestic violence as effectively as the classroom-based programme.

Another randomised controlled trial looked at a multidimensional programme to improve practice in preventing chlamydia infections.[2] The programme lasted 11 months. Doctors who did the programme significantly improved their knowledge, skills and clinical care. However, the programme was complex and included interactive case studies, performance feedback and patient leaflets.

Three short web-based courses to increase the identification of skin cancers have been evaluated.[3-5] One of these courses was a randomised controlled trial with 46 participants.[5] All of the courses significantly increased learners' knowledge and skills.

A randomised controlled trial evaluated a year-long interactive internet-based course in palliative care.[1,6] There were 179 participants and the study was performed in Finland. No significant change in treatment decisions and attitudes between the intervention and control groups was shown but the intervention group were more satisfied with their work.

In three studies the authors looked at user perspectives.[1,4,7] In these studies the authors reported high user satisfaction (especially related to flexibility, ease of access and efficiency).

The use of CD-ROMs

We identified two studies that evaluated self-instructional programmes on CD-ROMs.[8,9] One programme was about listening to heart murmurs[2,8] and the other was about management of cancer pain.[9] In both studies the learners who did the programmes showed significantly increased knowledge and skills. These studies were not randomised controlled trials.

The use of collaborative learning technology

We found 12 studies that evaluated the use of technology that enables collaborative learning. The technology was designed to provide opportunities for interactive discussions between colleagues. Seven studies used an online discussion group or email to facilitate interaction, and five studies used interactive videoconferencing.

Use of online discussion groups or email

Five studies described the use of collaborative learning technology in continuing professional development. Each study used a different approach. One randomised controlled trial looked at problem-based learning groups for the management of depression in the elderly.[10] The active group participated in a facilitated online discussion group, supported by a facilitator and two consultant psychiatrists, in addition to receiving learning resources. The control group was given similar learning resources via the internet but no interaction. The evaluation did not identify a difference in learning between the two groups.

However, in another study, the combined use of a CD-ROM, a web-based delivery system and an online discussion group improved learners' knowledge and skills.[11]

One study evaluated a facilitated online discussion group that was linked to an online course on diabetes: improved patient care was identified in addition to improvements in the learners' knowledge. The participants considered that the online discussion groups related well to their learning styles and fitted in with their time constraints. They also appreciated the opportunity to share information with colleagues and to work at their own pace.[12]

Participants in another study stated a preference for a structured approach with a facilitator.[13] This request for structure was also found in a study of access to conference facilities on an open-access continuing medical education website.[14]

Another study evaluated the use of email as an alternative to an online discussion group.[15] Learners who used email showed increased learning outcomes over time but no control group was used in the study.

Two studies evaluated the use of collaborative learning technology in programmes for training future general practitioners.[16,17] One study evaluated a virtual interactive seminar on nutrition with positive results,[16] and another study noted increased attendance at a series of interactive lectures while working at sites remote from the main institution.[17] Problems associated with providing this type of learning included technical difficulties and the fact that doctors needed time to adjust to the new approach.

Use of interactive videoconferencing

We found five studies that evaluated the use of interactive videoconferencing for small groups of general practitioners in remote and rural areas.[18–22] One study using a facilitated group noted that this approach was accepted well by users and that the users gained knowledge as a result.[22] Users in another study appreciated the reduced need to travel.[21] However, all studies commented on the associated technical difficulties, with several studies noting the wishes of participants to continue face-to-face meetings.

The use of information technology for education: attitudes and skills

We found nine studies that looked at attitudes to the use of information technology for education and whether users had the skills to be able to do it properly.[23–29] Doctors' confidence in the use of computers increased over time,[26] but both established general practitioners and those in training identified the need to develop their knowledge and skills.[23,24] Two studies identified lack of funding and time as the main barriers to meeting these learning needs.[25,27] Two studies found that the main use that general practitioners made of the internet was searching for information that was to be used for immediate patient care rather than taking part in online collaborative learning.[14,28] The use of information technology as a method to deliver continuing professional development was the least preferred option: the reason for this is that most doctors said that they didn't know how to do it.[29]

Discussion

We attempted to obtain a pragmatic review of the literature so that it would inform decision making, rather than an exhaustive systematic review. We recognise that there were some limitations in our approach to finding the literature, with articles on medical education being widely dispersed across numerous non-medical journals. However, our experience of reading literature in these journals suggested that our search strategy would be sufficient for the scope of the review. Information gathering was also hindered by the lack of recognition of the terms 'e-learning' and 'general practitioner' in the search vocabulary of Medline and Embase. However, we used a wide search strategy to maximise inclusion. The MeSH term 'computers' includes all specific terms that are related to personal computers, personal digital assistants, CD-ROMs and knowledge and attitudes to computers. The MeSH term 'computer communication networks' includes all discussion activities and the term 'electronic mail' includes the internet and email. The MeSH terms 'education, medical' and 'education, distance' were chosen for similar reasons. We were interested in e-learning within a healthcare context similar to the UK and only articles that described a primary care physician with a similar role to a general practitioner in the UK were included.

The majority of the identified studies were performed in the USA and Canada, with a few additional studies on interactive videoconferencing from Australia. Only two studies were identified that were performed in the United Kingdom.[7,13]

Studies were not formally assessed for methodological quality but we noted a general lack of high quality evidence. There were few randomised controlled trials and most studies included only small numbers of participants, typically less than 100.

Is it an effective method of education?

Evaluating the effectiveness of an educational intervention is a difficult concept but an important aspect is whether it produces a change in clinical or professional behaviour.[30] This is of particular importance to funding agencies. Only two studies were identified which demonstrated a change in clinical behaviour. In one study the educational intervention was complex and included feedback on performance, and in the other study the intervention included a combined online course and discussion group. However, most studies identified significant changes in the knowledge, skills and attitudes of participants. This change may be comparable to that achieved with a traditional classroom approach.

What methods are more effective?

No studies were identified that compared different methods of e-learning.

What are the opinions of learners?

Learners who participated in the studies were generally positive in their perceptions of e-learning. They valued the opportunity to share experiences with other colleagues and to be able to work at a pace that allowed self-directed learning. Rural general practitioners especially valued e-learning opportunities. In the USA, Canada and Australia there are major difficulties in providing outreach learning opportunities to isolated general practitioners but this may not be as applicable to the United Kingdom where there is less geographical isolation.

What are the barriers to implementation?

Most studies identified technological problems. Many learners stated that they had low competence in the use of information technology and that they needed time to adjust to this new form of learning. These findings are similar to those found in studies of general practitioners in the United Kingdom.[27]

Conclusion

Important lessons about e-learning for general practitioners have been identified but there is an urgent need for further published evaluations and research to improve the evidence base on which to inform future developments and policy decisions.

References

1 Harris JM, Kutob RM, Surprenant ZJ *et al.* (2002) Can Internet-based education improve physician confidence in dealing with domestic violence? *Family Medicine.* **34**: 107–12.
2 Casebeer LL, Strasser SM, Spettell CM *et al.* (2003) Designing tailored Web-based instruction to improve practising physician's preventive practices. *Journal of Medical Internet Research.* **5**: e20.
3 Pagnanelli G, Soyer HP, Argenziano G *et al.* (2003) Diagnosis of pigmented skin lesions

by dermoscopy: web-training improves diagnostic performance of non-experts. *British Journal of Dermatology.* **48**: 698–702.

4 Harris JM, Salasche SJ, Harris RB (2001) Can Internet-based continuing medical education improve physicians' skin cancer knowledge and skills. *Journal of General Internal Medicine.* **16**: 50–56.

5 Gerbert B, Bronstone A, Maurer T *et al.* (2002) The effectiveness of an Internet-based tutorial in improving primary care physicians' skin cancer triage skills. *Journal of Cancer Education.* **17**: 7–11.

6 Hinkka H, Kosunen E, Metsanoja R *et al.* (2002) General practitioners' attitudes and ethical decisions in end-of-life care after a year of interactive Internet-based training. *Journal of Cancer Education.* **17**: 12–18.

7 Agius RM and Bagnall G (1998) Development and evaluation of the use of the Internet as an educational tool in occupational and environmental health and medicine. *Occupational Medicine.* **48**: 337–43.

8 Roy D, Sargeant J, Gray J *et al.* (2002) Helping family physicians improve their cardiac auscultation skills with an interactive CD-ROM. *Journal of Continuing Education for Health Professionals.* **22**: 152–9.

9 Thompson AR, Savidge MA, Fulper-Smith M *et al.* (1999) Testing a multi-media module in cancer pain management. *Journal of Cancer Education.* **14**: 161–3.

10 Chan DH, Leclair K and Kaczorowski J (1999) Problem-based small group learning via the Internet among community family physicians: a randomised controlled trial. *MD Computing.* **16**: 54–8.

11 Curran VR, Hoekman T, Gullivar W *et al.* (2000) Web-based continuing medical education. (II): Evaluation study of computer-mediated continuing medical education. *Journal of Continuing Education for Health Professionals.* **20**: 106–19.

12 Wiecha J and Barrie N (2002) Collaborative online learning: a new approach to distance CME. *Academic Medicine.* **5**: 756–7.

13 Roberts C and Fox N (1998) General practitioners and the Internet: modelling a 'virtual community'. *Family Practice.* **15:** 211–15.

14 Dickmann C, Habermeyer E and Spitzer K (2000) WWW based continuing medical education: how do general practitioners use it? *Studies in Health Technology and Information.* **77**: 588–92.

15 Marshall JN, Stewart M and Ostbye T (2001) Small group CME using e-mail discussions. Can it work? *Canadian Family Physician.* **47**: 557–63.

16 Kolasa K, Poehlman G and Jobe A (2000) Virtual seminars for disseminating medical nutrition education curriculum ideas. *American Journal of Clinical Nutrition.* **71**: 1403–4.

17 Markova T and Roth LM (2002) E-conferencing for delivery of residency didactic. *Academic Medicine.* **77**: 748–9.

18 Sen Gupta TK, Wallace DA, Clark SL *et al.* (1998) Videoconferencing: practical advice on implementation. *Australian Journal of Rural Health.* **6**: 2–4.

19 Calla M, Ricci MA and Caputo MP (2000) Improved rural provider access to continuing medical education through interactive videoconferencing. *Telemedicine Journal.* **6**: 393–9.

20 Davis P and McCracken P (2002) Restructuring rural continuing medical education through videoconferencing. *Journal of Telemedicine and Telecare.* **8**: 108–9.

21 Allen M, Sargeant J, MacDougall E *et al.* (2002) Videoconferencing for continuing medical education: from pilot project to sustained programme. *Journal of Telemedicine and Telecare.* **8**: 131–7.

22 Allen M, Sargeant J, Mann K *et al.* (2003) Videoconferencing for practice-based small group continuing medical education: feasibility, acceptability, effectiveness and cost. *Journal of Continuing Education for Health Professionals.* **23**: 38–47.

23 Cook MC, Hartman JA and Russell LR (1998) Integrating personal computers into family practice: a comparison of practising physicians and residents. *Bulletin of the Medical Librarians Association.* **86**: 316–25.

24 McClaran J, Snell L and Duarte-Franco E (2000) Continuing educational needs in computers and information. McGill survey of family physicians. *Canadian Family Physician.* **46**: 839–47.
25 Jerant AF and Lloyd AJ (2000) Applied medical informatics and computing skills of students, residents and faculty. *Family Medicine.* **32**: 267–72.
26 Jerant AF, Matian AD and Lasslo RG (2003) Increases in resident and faculty computing skills between 1998 and 2001. *Family Medicine.* **35**: 202–8.
27 Wilson SM (1999) Impact of the Internet on primary care staff in Glasgow. *Journal of Medical Internet Research.* **1**: 1.
28 Casebeer LL, Bennett N, Kristofco R *et al.* (2002) Physician Internet medical information seeking and on-line continuing education use patterns. *Journal of Continuing Education for Health Professionals.* **22**: 33–42.
29 Mamary EM and Charles P (2000) On-site to on-line: barriers to the use of computers for continuing education. *Journal of Continuing Education in the Health Professions.* **20**: 171–5.
30 Kirkpatrick DL (1998) *Evaluating Training Programs: the four levels.* Berrett-Koehler, San Francisco.

Chapter 3

A personal experience of using e-learning

David Bossano

Key points

- A major attraction of e-learning is its flexibility.
- There are several approaches to e-learning, both formal and informal.
- An essential part of e-learning is the opportunity to enter a discussion with colleagues.
- Practice-based email offers a useful method for learning.

Introduction

I will start with a recent scenario as an illustration of my use of e-learning and I will return to it at the end of the chapter. Jack is an African man, the same age as me. He came in to see me because the attack of shingles that started three days ago seems to be getting worse, even though my colleague started aciclovir in the first hours. He is otherwise well and there is no evidence of secondary infection.

The alarm bells are ringing. His partner is in Africa, he doesn't know if she has HIV/AIDs. I explain that we need to check him out for this. The problem is, our practice's historical policy is that we always refer people who need HIV testing. The waiting list for the GUM clinic is long. The infectious disease clinic is 5 miles away. Jack is an asylum seeker and has little cash in hand.

I take the blood myself and ask him to come back two days later. The result is positive. We talk about the implications. I refer him to the next clinic at the local hospital. At least his shingles has improved with simple analgesia and completing the aciclovir.

Later I email my colleagues. A new case of HIV. A GP has been on a sexual health course. Shingles in a young adult equals HIV. A nurse practitioner has worked in a GUM clinic. We aren't testing enough people. Another GP works with drug users, we should consider testing for Hepatitis C and other blood-borne viruses a lot more readily. Following this email discussion we discuss this at a practice meeting. We agree to consider testing for HIV more readily than in the past and a small working group investigates the implications for the practice.

My background

I have been an inner city GP in Manchester for five years. The above scenario happens with variations most weeks. The practice is large and busy but I am fortunate to have enthusiastic and interested colleagues, and wonderful patients. We have a meeting once a week but most days, we only have a chance to smile and wave in the corridor.

My partner is also a GP. We have a three-year-old daughter and our son is due now. We both work part-time and do childcare. Personal study has to be fitted in around these commitments, often late at night or during children's naps.

Before coming to Manchester we worked for two years in Papua New Guinea as VSO medical officers. Our work mainly involved supporting and training primary healthcare workers and the materials we used were books and chalk boards. Although e-learning has its place, the majority of people in the world are probably still unable to benefit from it.

When I returned to the UK I had to update my practice and it seemed that quite a lot had changed while I'd been away. I used computerised records for the first time and everyone had a mobile phone. I enrolled on various postgraduate courses and over the last few years have had a range of learning experiences.

My own use of e-learning

I have been studying on the web-based Masters in Population Health Evidence (MPHe) degree programme for the past three years. I have also used the BMJlearning website on many occasions. At work I share problems with colleagues by internal email. I have used a variety of other online resources over the last few years. The NeLH (National Electronic Library for Health www.nelh.nhs. uk/) is my favourite portal and has useful links to many other resources, including PubMed, Bandolier, Prodigy etc. My practice changed computer system to EMIS PCS a year ago and recently I have come to use EMIS Webmentor® more frequently.

The MPHe programme

This is based entirely online (www.mphe.man.ac.uk). It consists of a number of modules and the content of each of each module is available online during the semester it is taken. Each module is divided into sections of roughly a week's work. Every section briefly covers a topic and also contains many links to other learning materials on the internet. 'Seminars' are held in the form of a facilitated discussion board, to which a small group of students taking that module contribute. Course work is also submitted electronically.

The good things were the flexibility of the course materials and discussion, which could be accessed any time; the course material provided an excellent overview and links to many online resources. The discussion boards enabled sharing and developing of learning.

The downside was that in some areas all the information was provided in the form of links and that the discussion boards didn't always 'take off'.

BMJ learning

This consists of online tutorials on a wide range of topics (www.bmjlearning.com). The materials I have used have contained an up-to-date, practical summary of that topic area. There is a self-test at the end: a record for one's PDP.

Again, it is very flexible in that it can be accessed at any time. The material is excellent.

The negatives for me were that the materials I used didn't have links to other online resources and there was no opportunity to interact/discuss with the author or other learners.

Work-based email

There are around 25 clinicians at The Robert Darbishire Practice and there are limited opportunities to interact and discuss cases face to face. Instead we make use of internal email to address a wide range of queries and other issues. Areas covered include clinical, practical, ethical and legal problems, resources and information. Responses allow sharing of uncertainty and providing support. They can include quick advice or refer to online and other resources.

The strengths of work-based email include its convenience and flexibility. Responses tend to be practical and there is a selection to compare and choose from. Email discussions enable attitudes to change as well as knowledge. The main drawback is that responses are personal and subjective.

The strengths of e-learning

The main advantage of e-learning for me is its flexibility, allowing me to fit learning around a busy practice and family life. It allows me to access a regularly updated summary of a topic and this is enhanced by links to a huge range of other online resources. It may provide a forum for discussion.

Areas where e-learning could be developed further

Deep learning arises from interaction (between learners and between the learner and the subject).

Interaction allows attitudes to be developed as well as knowledge and possibly skills. Interaction may work best in a relatively small group of colleagues who know and trust each other. Facilitating interaction in a group who don't know each other or who have very different roles, appears harder.

My observations of work-based email as a form of e-learning

I recently undertook a study at work to analyse the use of email to support learning and change of practice. I used a practitioner-based method that had the aim of describing who participated in the use of email and what was discussed. Emails were collected opportunistically over a six-month period and analysed to investigate what was covered, who took part, what was learnt and how this compared to other possible forms of learning or changing practice.

I analysed 68 emails and discovered that these generally involved all the GPs, practice nurses and nurse practitioner, and sometimes included the practice manager and secretarial staff, particularly when related to significant event discussion or issues about keeping patients on the list. The areas covered were broad and included useful resources, interesting papers and the availability of new services and clinics. Other topics arose from patient contacts and could be divided into roughly eight distinct areas, which were: results (interpretation and management e.g. isolated raised alkaline phosphatase); management (e.g. phantom limb pain); referral (is there a service and how do I refer to it e.g. hypnotherapy); therapeutics (interactions e.g. clopidogrel and warfarin); ethical/professional dilemmas (e.g. response to alteration of sick note or prescription, patient declines referral for sinister symptoms); clinical governance (significant event audits/near misses e.g. failure to act on a positive test result); support (e.g. late diagnosis of cancer in someone who refused referral for worrying symptoms); and finally hypothesis generation (e.g. there have been five cases of cancer in under-30s: is it a cluster?). Many of these topics could stimulate learning, both individual and within the practice team.

Back to my initial scenario

There are many aspects of this scenario which could prompt a search for different online resources.

For example, I could have looked for the benefit of aciclovir in reducing the duration and pain of shingles. Excellent resources are the Cochrane Library or Clinical Evidence, both accessible via NeLH. Or I could have looked up information about the likelihood of developing overt HIV in a young adult with shingles by using 'PubMed Clinical Queries – Prognosis', also available via NeLH.

However, for me, the greatest impact on my learning and change in practice has come from discussions with colleagues, which has in my workplace been facilitated by the use of email discussion.

Conclusion

e-learning is not a fundamentally different form of learning. Deep learning (i.e. change in behaviour) probably depends on interaction with learning material and with people. New technology enables this interaction to happen electronically at a time, pace and usually a place that is convenient for the learner. e-learning resources allow links to vast amounts of information but new knowledge requires the added experience of trusted colleagues and this requires the opportunity to enter into peer discussion.

Chapter 4

The challenge of e-learning for GP educators

John Sandars and Michele Langlois

Key points

- The majority of GP educators frequently used websites for personal use and for personal learning.
- Chat rooms and discussion lists were rarely used by GP educators for either personal use or for personal learning.
- GP educators were unsure how to fit e-learning in with their present role as an educator.
- The use of e-learning in GP education has yet to find its place and is a challenge to all GP educators.

Introduction

There can be no doubt that e-learning will become an increasingly important part of the provision of all medical education, including education in primary care, over the next few years. The future direction of education in primary care will be determined by major initiatives that are the result of the Government's education, National Health Service (NHS) and technological agendas.[1]

It is not expected, or likely, that many educators in primary care will develop e-learning materials, such as online course or CD-ROMs, since these require highly specific skills. However, all educators will need the knowledge and skills to enable all learners to maximise their use of the available e-learning opportunities. This will become increasingly important as more core educational content is electronically delivered. There will be several new activities for educators, depending on their individual roles. First, they will need to guide learners to appropriate e-learning resources for self-study, perhaps as part of meeting learning needs identified by problem-based methods or personal development plans (PDPs). Second, they will need to integrate e-learning resources into current educational activities, such as day release courses, an approach called 'blended learning'. The impact of e-learning on vocational training and continuing professional development (CPD) in primary care will depend on how trainers, course organisers and CPD tutors respond to this new challenge.

The results of a recent survey of e-learning by GP educators

We recently performed an in-magazine questionnaire survey of the readers of *Education for Primary Care* (November 2003) in an attempt to identify how information technology and e-learning is used for personal use by educators in primary care, and also in their role as an educator. Despite a low response rate (107 completed questionnaires, 7.4%), which is typical of similar surveys,[2] the results offer a useful insight into the challenges that need to be met by educators in primary care.

Socio-demographic characteristics of the respondents

A slightly higher proportion of males responded and just over half were aged between 40 and 49 years. Most were trainers or course organisers, with 14% GP tutors for CPD the remainder.

Use of information technology (IT)

The majority of respondents (70%) regularly used the internet at least weekly for obtaining information. Only two of the respondents had never used the internet but 18% used it daily. Over three-quarters had never used chat rooms or discussion lists for personal use.

Use of e-learning for personal learning

Similar numbers of respondents used the internet for personal learning as those for obtaining information for other reasons. The use of specialised medical databases, such as Medline, to support work was still popular whilst slightly less often used. Only 3% never used medical databases but 70% had used them at least once a month for their own personal learning: 15% of respondents stated that they had studied on a web-based distance learning course. These were from a variety of suppliers but most were clinical topics supplied by commercial organisation. Only two stated that they had undertaken a higher degree programme by distance learning. Chat rooms and discussion lists were slightly more popular for personal learning reasons but were still underutilised, although 64% had never used them and 7% used them at least once a week.

Attitudes towards e-learning resources

The majority of respondents (80%) held positive attitudes on the use of e-learning resources compared with other resources. Several commented on their experience of using e-learning resources (including the internet, CD-ROMs and web-based learning courses) to support their work. Several themes emerged from these comments, as the following excerpts illustrate:

> The information is often more up to date and saves time by not going to the library. Local resources may not have the info required.

Knowing what to use is difficult – so much info that could waste a lot of time.

Still find it impossible (or at least unpleasant!) to read long comments online. Broadband availability at home has made a big difference (even if it means doing more work at home!).

Overall, there was an appreciation of the ease of accessibility but there were also frustrations with problems related the time required to access information. These difficulties were stated to be due not only to the technology but to lack of skills and unfamiliarity with the electronic medium.

Use of e-learning resources in activities as an educator

A total of 80% of respondents replied that they used e-learning resources in their activities as an educator, with most (85%) using them at least monthly. The most commonly stated were the internet (53%), specific medical websites (31%), CD-ROMs (27%) and electronic databases such as Medline (15%). Only six stated that they thought e-learning resources were of little or no use in their activities as an educator. The majority (84%) indicated that they intended to use e-learning resources in their activities as an educator in the future, with 64 stating that they definitely would. Only 10 were undecided.

The most commonly stated advantages of e-learning were current information, the quickness and ease of access to a wide range of resources. It was also stated that e-learning allowed the learner to work at their own pace. Only 10% of respondents noted that e-learning provided an opportunity to interact with others. The main disadvantages were related to difficulties in technology and access, information overload, variable quality of information, time required and lack of skills. Two respondents stated that they hated computers and needed to change their habits. Being unsure how to fit it in with their present role as an educator was noted by several respondents, with one stating that they required more training on the potential uses of e-learning in education. Some examples of respondents' attitudes reflecting these themes are provided below.

Advantages

Accessibility in different locations. Fit with my and registrar's learning style – immediate ability to look up and save interesting things. More likely to get access to the patient experience.

Ability to search different sources/databases. Share ideas and gain feedback. Allow questions to be asked after a session. Often up to date. Extends the learning time.

The material tends to be more up to date. Format tends to be more interesting. You often browse into other areas of interest.

Disadvantages

> Can be distracting as it is so much fun. If the PC crashes I can't access it. Sometimes too much information to scan but this is better if I use training websites.

> Too difficult to read off a computer screen. Easy to get distracted and follow red herrings online and lose track of time.

> Often takes a long time to find what you want. Need to filter out irrelevant search material. Non-academic pages may be non-evidence-based and biased by specific interests.

> No substitute for good books in some areas. Good on knowledge not good on skills except typing.

Correlations between categories

There was a significant negative correlation between the use of websites for personal use and age. There were no significant differences according to sex or occupation. There were significant positive correlations between the use of websites to obtain information for personal use and both the use of websites to support work and with the perceived usefulness of e-learning resources for personal use.

Discussion

It is important to consider the results of this survey in relation to other studies. The majority of respondents frequently used websites for personal use and for personal learning. The use of e-learning for personal learning was considered to be useful but respondents identified several difficulties, especially accessibility of technology and lack of time and skills. These difficulties have also been identified in two surveys of UK general practices and their use of the internet and NHSnet.[3,4]

Chat rooms and discussion lists were rarely used for either personal use or for personal learning. This method of communication has the potential to increase social interaction, and collaborative learning, between professionals who are at a distance from each other.[5] The importance of online collaborative learning as a method of continuing professional development has only recently been emphasised as a method of e-learning.[6] Most web-based distance learning courses only offer a one-to-one relationship between the computer and the learner. Several respondents stated that their experience of online collaborative learning was positive, with sharing of best practice and knowledge within a field of interest, but they also noted that it was hampered by poor involvement of group participants and lengthy, tedious discussions. Similar difficulties have been noted before in the UK with general practitioners online.[7]

The significant correlations between the use of websites for personal use, such as obtaining information for non-work related use and the use of websites to obtain information to support work and the perceived usefulness of e-learning resources for personal learning, suggest that educators who used the internet for personal use are more likely to have used it for personal learning. It was interesting to note the presence of 'computerphobia' in some of the educators in primary care, with avoidance of the use of computers.[8] This is not a skills issue but relates to an attitude to the use of computers.

This survey was the first reported from the UK and probably represented a subset with high interest and commitment to e-learning. They can be regarded as 'trendsetters' or early adopters.[9] Overall, this survey identified that there is an overall appreciation of the value of e-learning for education in primary care, with many educators having personal experience of e-learning. This enthusiasm was also apparent in their role as an educator. However, the survey also identified many difficulties that are associated with this new role. These can be considered within a framework than covers competencies, connectivity and content.[10]

Competencies

This includes the development of skills, not only in the use of information technology such as basic computer skills and working with information, but also how to use the variety of new e-learning opportunities in their role as a GP educator. There are early initiatives by the NHS Information Authority to increase training in the basic skills for all healthcare staff, but all GP educators will need to become more confident and competent in these areas as the ability of the NHS workforce increases.

Connectivity

This includes the technical aspects of accessing the information through computer systems. The NHSnet may be widespread but there may still be difficulties with inter-operability between different systems and e-learning providers, including difficulties in access due to NHSnet security features and poor home access to the internet, including lack of broadband availability. All educators in primary care will need to be aware of these difficulties, both to support learners who are experiencing problems, but also to work with local e-learning strategy groups which will be responsible for implementing e-learning.

Content

This includes the educational quality of the learning content that is provided. It has been emphasised that high quality e-learning should be based on sound adult learning principles, to ensure that there is interaction between the learner and the content, learning is linked to work experiences, learning is supported by experienced tutors and learners have the opportunity to interact with other learners.[11] This will require all GP educators to be skilled in evaluating the quality of the learning content and delivery, enabling them to make informed choices about using these materials in their teaching and in their recommendations to learners. e-learning includes a wide variety of educational resources, with a range from self-study instructional materials, such as CD-ROMs, to online collaborative learning networks. It is important that this breadth is fully appreciated by educators and that opportunities are identified in current, and future, educational activities to allow this medium to be fully utilised.

The future place of e-learning in GP education is uncertain but this is typical of any new technology being introduced in education. Edward Lias has commented on the overall impact of new technology,[12] and he presents several points that are useful to consider. First, there is an increasing spiral of dependency following the introduction of any new technology. Once something new is introduced it creates new uses for itself and it is expected that more e-learning approaches will become available, rather than less. Second, embedded in any new technology is an underlying philosophy, but this may be not be readily apparent, with the consequence that change may occur without adequate discussion and understanding of the consequences. An important consideration for all GP educators is the nature of the underlying educational philosophy of the new e-learning approach. The relationship between educators and new technology has been noted by Larry Cuban as always being a 'fickle romance'.[13] Film and radio were introduced in the 1920s and 1930s, television in the 1950s and 1960s, and computers from the 1970s. He observed that each new technology was heralded as a way to revolutionalise education, with the promise of more effective and efficient learning, but the reality has been that each technology has been followed by disillusionment. He noted that academic studies have usually only documented small learning effects from each new technology and that the consequence has been that there was a never-ending search for newer technology to deliver learning content. It has never been a more important time for all GP educators to effectively respond to the challenge and develop their knowledge.

Recommendations for future development and policy

We recommend that action is required to increase the confidence and competence of all GP educators in the use of IT, working with information and in using e-learning in their provision of education. It is suggested that a systematic process is undertaken, including the following:

- Develop a core competency framework for e-learning skills that is applicable to all GP educators. This requires that the core skills should be identified and collated to develop a national standard.
- Perform a training needs analysis for e-learning skills in all GP educators. This will allow the assessment of the extent of e-learning skills so that the training needs can be identified.
- Develop a training programme to increase the e-learning skills of all GP educators in primary care. This will need to be based on the identified learning needs.

Conclusion

It has never been a more important time for all GP educators to effectively respond to the challenge of e-learning. It is essential that they develop their knowledge, skills and awareness of the e-learning approach to GP education otherwise the full potential of e-learning may not be realised and, at its worst, the future of GP education may be put in jeopardy.

Acknowledgments

We would like to thank the respondents to the questionnaire that was sent with the November 2003 issue of *Education for Primary Care*.

References

1 Sandars J (2003) e-learning: the coming of age. *Education for Primary Care.* **14**: 1–5.
2 Brennan M (1992) Techniques for improving mail survey response rates. *Marketing Bulletin.* **3**: 24–37.
3 Wilson SM (1999) Impact of the Internet on primary care staff in Glasgow. *Journal of Medical Internet Research.* **1**: 1.
4 Wilson P, Glanville J and Watt I (2003) Access to the online evidence base in general practice: a survey of the Northern and Yorkshire Region. *Health Information and Library Journal.* **20**: 172–8.
5 Anderson T and Kanuka H (1997) On-line forums: new platforms for professional development and group collaboration. *Journal of Computer Mediated Communication.* **3**: 1–15.
6 Wiecha J and Barrie N (2002) Collaborative online learning: a new approach to distance CME. *Academic Medicine.* **5**: 756–7.
7 Roberts C and Fox N (1998) General practitioners and the Internet: modelling a 'virtual community'. *Family Practice.* **15**: 211–15.
8 Jay T (1981) Computerphobia. What to do about it. *Educational Technology.* **21**: 47–8.
9 Solomon MB (1996) Targeting trendsetters. *Marketing Research.* **8**: 9–11.
10 Library and Information Commission (2003) *2020 Vision.* Library and Information Commission, London.
11 Institute for Higher Education Policy (2000) *Quality On the Line.* Institute for Higher Education Policy, Washington, DC.
12 Lias EJ (1982) *Future Mind.* Little Brown, Boston.
13 Cuban L (1986) *Teachers and Machines: the classroom use of technology since 1920.* Teachers College Press, New York.

Chapter 5

The educational foundations of e-learning for healthcare professionals

Andrew Thornett and Rachel Davey

Key points

- The emphasis of e-learning has changed from information transfer to information processing.
- Virtual Learning Environments can provide an overall structure to learning activities and opportunities.
- Effective e-learning recognises the importance of learning styles and attempts to provide a range of learning activities.
- Discussion forums and virtual classrooms can provide interaction between students.
- An important aspect of e-learning is the development of communities of practice.

Introduction

Traditionally, education in healthcare has been didactic or involved learning practical skills at the patient's bedside, with the aim of creating professionals who demonstrate the same modes of thinking and knowledge base as their teachers. This style of education was appropriate when treatment protocols and guidelines changed little over time and whilst the evidence base for treatment was poor with few effective treatments available. However, in the current environment, the health professional is faced with a rapidly evolving evidence base for a portfolio of increasingly effective treatments. Treating according to the research evidence base is seen as an important aspect of good healthcare practice,[1,2] but cannot be done without the skills to search and critically review the literature. The modern health practitioner must also be able to take into account uncertainty and risk in his or her assessments, diagnosis and choice of management strategies,[3–5] and be aware of political realities and the possibility of litigation.

This chapter explores the role of e-learning in meeting these emerging needs and explores such modes of delivery in the light of learning theory for health professionals. Examples are provided from our own experience of delivering e-learning postgraduate courses and continuing professional development (CPD) within the Faculty of Health and Sciences at Staffordshire University using Blackboard™ (www.blackboard.com/) a web-based Virtual Learning Environment

(VLE), which allows students to access learning material from any computer with internet access. Students can conduct their learning activities, collaborate and access resources away from the lecture room. Students generally find the system easy to navigate. Information is provided in a number of folder areas: course information, staff information, course documents, assignments, communication etc.

The education needs of new roles for health professionals

Health professionals in many discipline groups are taking on new roles that take them into territories not previously explored by their predecessors. This is seen at its most extreme in nursing and allied health practice, where the traditional roles of doctors are now increasingly being performed by professionals without primary medical training. The result of differences in disciplinary background between teachers and students and between students means that the traditional apprenticeship model of training fails to address the needs of current student cohorts. Teachers must instead look for alternative ways of helping them to develop into effective and safe practitioners.

Part of the answer can be found in new educational methods that incorporate decision making at a higher level in the curriculum – changing the emphasis from information transfer to information processing. The rapidly increasing use of problem-based learning (PBL) methods in the curriculum is indicative here.

Probably of more importance is the emphasis upon lifelong learning for professionals in healthcare. This involves reflection upon personal work in order to determine learning needs for the future. For many practitioners, this requires the development of new skills in critical review and analysis that will allow them to integrate the evolving evidence base into their existing knowledge. These skills incorporate the ability to judge the quality of research evidence and to apply it in personal practice.

There has been much debate about the best mode of delivery to use to meet these new educational needs. Traditional modes of face-to-face delivery and distance learning using paper-based methods fall foul of the professionals' need to access materials that respond and change depending on current priorities within the healthcare environment. The former requires their attendance at an educational centre that is often at distance from the workplace, requires time off work and carries expensive overheads for buildings and educators. The latter lacks some of the social components of learning and the benefits that can be gained by hearing colleagues' experiences and suggestions. In comparison, online courses can be accessible all day every day, and student interaction with colleagues and tutors is an important component for a large part of that time.

e-learning and blended e-learning

e-learning has been seen by many as the solution to these problems. It allows materials to be actively and rapidly changed to reflect the learning base, can be accessed from within the environment in which the professional practices, and does not require the large overhead of face-to-face courses. Unlike paper-based packages, students can also interact with each other in the online environment using the discussion forum. Learning sets and groups can be mimicked within this setting.

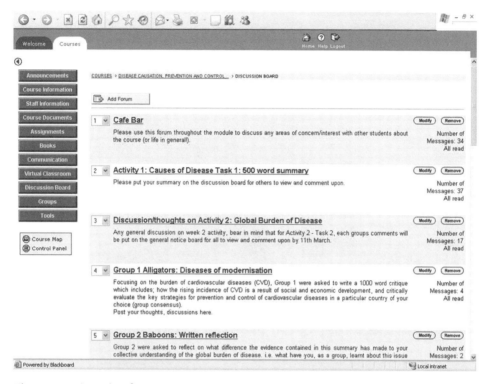

Figure 5.1 Discussion forums

We use 'blended' e-learning which integrates a combination of online course content written in Word documents with web-based online hyperlinks. Students have direct access to the World Wide Web (WWW) which provides a whole range of resources that supplement and broaden the learning experience by using a variety of resources (blended into course content). These resources include electronic journals, e-books, key websites and databases, and allow students to access online information at their own pace and in their own time. The main idea behind blended learning is that instructional designers review a learning programme, break it up into smaller units (modules) and determine the best medium to deliver these modules to the learner.

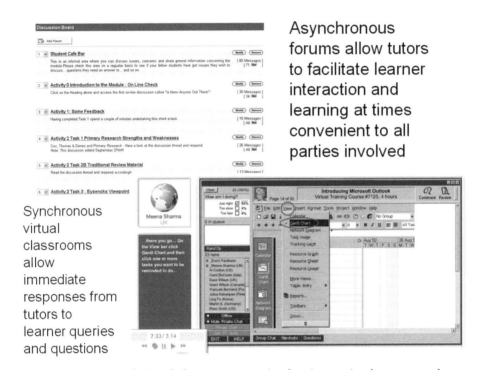

Asynchronous forums allow tutors to facilitate learner interaction and learning at times convenient to all parties involved

Synchronous virtual classrooms allow immediate responses from tutors to learner queries and questions

Figure 5.2 Forums and virtual classrooms can stimulate interaction between students

What can the experiential learning cycle teach us about e-learning?

Ausubel in 1960 pointed out how important it was to ensure that learners understood concepts in terms of their own experiences and previous understanding.[6] It is also important for educators to address learners' preferred learning styles when designing e-learning opportunities.

A number of authors have identified preferred learning styles for many individuals. These differ between professionals and between teachers and their students and can affect the learning experience in order to improve the learning that occurs or to limit its effectiveness. One of the most famous learning style questionnaires has been developed by Honey and Mumford.[7,8]

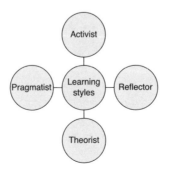

Figure 5.3 Honey and Mumford's four learning styles

For each of us, our learning style relates most closely to a particular part of the Kolb cycle[9] and it is this aspect of learning that we find most easy and intuitive. Nevertheless, whatever our preference, in order to learn effectively we all need to go completely around the cycle. In the first stage of this cycle, planning and preparing, a learner identifies an important gap in his or her knowledge or skills required for his or her profession, and determines learning needs; i.e. between present and desired states of knowledge or skills. Kolb then described the need for the learner to work out what is needed to move from one state to the other, to understand the signs that signal that this move has occurred, and then plan to undertake an appropriate activity to fulfil that learning need. In the second stage, the learner must engage in this learning activity, and then, in the third stage,[10] reflect on the experience, in order to, finally, generalise and internalise the lessons from the experience. A comparison is again made between the new current state and the desired state of learning, and the results of this comparison lead to a further stage of preparing and planning.[11]

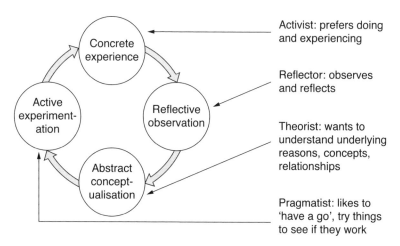

Figure 5.4 Honey and Mumford typology of learners

For educators, this means that if they direct their teaching towards the student's preferred learning style then the student will be most able to relate to the concepts and activities presented and be better able to integrate the learning into his or her professional life. As student groups in reality consist of individuals in all four categories above, in practice this means that educators should ensure that their teaching addresses the learning styles of the whole group. In addition, they should make efforts to assist the students to progress completely around the cycle.

The e-learning environment can assist the educator to achieve these aims. From the initial introduction to the VLE, the experience can be individualised for each student.

Electronic resources can store much larger amounts of information than paper-based resources, and the WWW provides an even greater information resource opportunity. If written well, web pages do not need to present this information all at once, but can allow students to access only those parts of interest to them. In addition, the content of web pages can change as a result of student's responses so

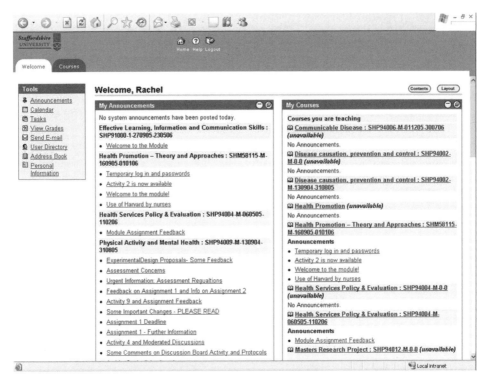

Figure 5.5 VLEs can personalise the student experience

that no two students view exactly the same information, targeting the learning experience to their preferred style. Increased interactivity is provided through student interaction or with their tutors either synchronously (at the same time) or asynchronously (at different times) using virtual classrooms or discussion forums.

Difficulties that may arise in addressing the needs of different learners in the online environment

Kolb identified four key skills for effective learning:

1   concrete experience abilities
2   reflective observation abilities
3   abstract conceptualisation abilities and
4   active experimentation abilities, which can be viewed as polar endpoints of two dimensions of learning: a concrete–abstract and active–reflective dimension.[12]

Not all learners possess these skills when they first experience online learning. In practice it is often difficult to get students to interact with each other virtually. Students' level of IT skills prior to commencing online learning has been shown to be important in explaining module completion and outcome.[10] Unfortunately, for many health professionals, their experience of e-learning will be the first they have ever undertaken and their IT skills and experience limited.

Additionally, fear and uncertainty are often experienced by individuals when initially accessing internet-based learning opportunities. This tends to lead to reluctance to get involved in all activities presented to them. As they are not in the classroom, learners lack the encouragement and positive feedback that having colleagues around them provides. However, once they have succeeded in overcoming this hurdle and begin to participate in the online activities, such interaction is available and encourages further interaction and success. This initial difficulty obtaining support can put many students off from continuing with their education in the online environment or from making best use of the technology. Educators need to be aware of the presence of this initial hurdle and ensure that appropriate induction procedures and education in IT is available at the start of the course to help learners over the problems that arise from its presence.

Other environmental considerations include slow or unreliable internet connections. When connections break or are slow, students may question why they chose this modality for their learning. Our students are given the minimum PC specification required before they register onto the course and are given free anti-virus software to help minimise these problems. Again, ideally educators should ensure that online material is accessible by learners whatever the connection speed or computer specification. It is probably best to avoid video or large pictures unless absolutely necessary or at least to ensure that they are not a core part of the curriculum and can be accessed in an alternative way if required (e.g. as a video ordered from the educational institution). Further, for some individuals, getting time off work is particularly important, and the use of an online system may mean that this is not forthcoming. Protected time allows students to concentrate on their studies and is particularly important when a subject is new or complex.

The other principal skills of reflection and critical review develop as the course progresses but may hinder initial interaction and application. It is worth providing links to appropriate sites or library material to enable students to explore these areas further as needed in their own homes and to bring up these topics in the discussion forums. Stating the problems openly in this way can prevent despair and depression when learners face the inevitable sense of loss and uncertainty that comes from new ideas and perspectives.

Active and collaborative learning

So where does e-learning stand out from other forms of information provision such as books or standard written distance learning courses?

Although intranet, internet or CD-ROM access can immediately link to a range of learning resources and information, the answer to this question lies in the medium's ability to provide active learning experiences via interactive and dynamic web content. Online learning experiences should seek to encourage the learner to enter a new virtual interactive environment, motivate them to stay there and then encourage them to take what they've learnt and apply it to their own professional work in the world outside.

Box 5.1 What the internet can offer for the learning experience

- Active knowledge construction.
- Increased understanding and ability to apply in real life when learners attempt to apply the knowledge they learn during the learning process.
- Achieved by:
  - links to a broader and more easily accessible knowledge
  - increased range of student interaction outside of the classroom
  - links to formative assessment activities.

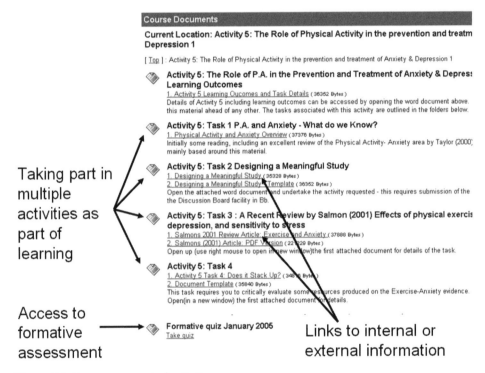

Figure 5.6 Encouragement of activity

Aspects of high quality e-learning provision that provide such experiences include those with a high level of interaction and supervision (*see* Figure 5.5), and where the learner can dip in and out of learning easily and regularly, as his or her professional learning needs dictate. Formative assessment can provide immediate feedback on students' progress and help them to ensure they are on the right track.

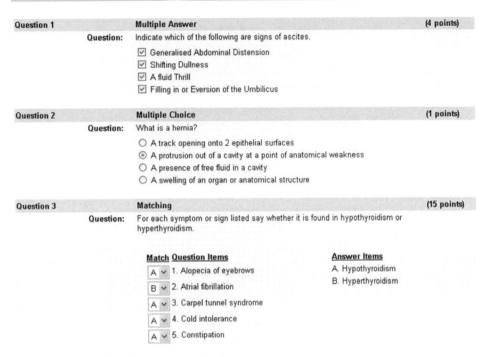

Figure 5.7 Providing formative feedback

Discussion forums and the development of a learning community

Constructivists approaches to learning and teaching promote the value of student discussions and collaborative working. Several communication modes are offered in Blackboard, giving students more flexibility in the methods they choose to communicate with staff and students. For example, direct email, the 'Announcement Board', asynchronous and synchronous discussion forums, and learning sets (usually between 6–8 students). Group leaders are assigned to co-ordinate their learning set's activities for various tasks required and to collate data and feedback to the main discussion forum. Learning sets are particularly useful if there are a large number of students on the module and where discussion gets too 'noisy' (each learning set only sees their own group's discussion). Learning sets can be given a different task/problem and asked to feedback their collective response to the main discussion forum.

Individual or group contributions to these discussions can be integrated into both summative and formative assessment and can give the tutor valuable feedback on how students are progressing (or not, as the case may be!).

One interesting observation with discussion forums, is that unlike face-to-face discussion, the student tends to think and reflect more upon statements presented. Rather than commenting on something 'off the top of their head' so to speak (as often occurs in face-to-face discussion), the student has more time to think and reflect carefully upon the comments that they would like to contribute and hence discussion tends to be of a higher quality.

Situating e-learning within its social context

A changing social environment also impacts upon the way people learn best. For Vygotsky, 'The development of an individual's skills, both subject specific and general, is intrinsically linked to the culture of the particular society and the learning activities which are shared within that context'.[13] We all learn within a particular socio-political context and none of us simply take in information but interpret and integrate it into our lives in a way that is acceptable and makes sense to us as members of the group in which we live and work. As practising health workers this is particularly important, as what we say and do needs to make sense to our patients as well as our colleagues, and, as educators, addressing this area for our students will mean they will be more open to the lessons taught and achieve better learning outcomes.

Online learning environments should ensure that this application is easy to achieve for learners by taking into account the real-life hurdles they will face to implement the lessons they've learnt in practice. The better the course, the more it will deal with these issues during the course, and the more likely the lessons are to make a difference to practice and this will lead to better retention of new knowledge and skills. In many cases, these issues are dealt with through feedback from colleagues and tutors in asynchronous or synchronous forums, enabling learners to apply knowledge learnt in practice by relating it to its social context during the learning process.

Feedback

The online environment provides an opportunity to provide formative feedback to learners, which can help prevent learners based at distance from the educational centre from losing their way in their studies. However, it is more difficult to demonstrate sensitivity and consideration online than face-to-face, and efforts need to be put into the wording of comments and advice as a result. Educators should not forget face-to-face meetings or the telephone – just because the course is mostly online doesn't mean that occasional extra efforts might not be required!

Particularly useful is the ability to conduct online formative assessments in VLEs. Automatic feedback can be given which can include links to further information or web resources. These assessments often work best in conjunction with an online forum in which students discuss their results and help each other to discover the answers – tutors need to feed into these forums but if care is taken you can give just enough information to stimulate group learning but not too much that you stifle it.

Conclusion

As educators of healthcare professionals we need to ensure that we use the most effective methods of delivering education at our disposal. If we are going to use e-learning then we need to ensure that we understand what its potential benefits are for health professionals, and the barriers they experience when they try to access material delivered this way in their professional work.

The VLE provides educators with an opportunity to provide learners with educational opportunities that are more than just a textbook on the web. Active and participatory learning allows learners to progress completely around Kolb's experiential learning cycle, reviewing new information and applying it to their own work as professionals through practical exercises. Feedback can be made available automatically from formative assessment systems, and from tutors and fellow learners via asynchronous and synchronous discussion forums and virtual classrooms. Online networks of like-minded professionals can be used to build communities of practice and learning that can build on initial experiences to enable learners to continue to improve and review their practice throughout their lives.

However, in many cases, the evidence underlying the effectiveness and cost-effectiveness of e-learning is poor and more effort needs to be made to improve this evidence through appropriate research and evaluation.

References

1 Gluud C and Gluud LL (2005) Evidence based diagnostics. *BMJ*. **330**: 724–6.
2 Department of Health (2005) Promoting implementation research findings. www.dh. gov.uk/PolicyAndGuidance/ResearchAndDevelopment/ResearchAndDevelopment AZ/PromotingImplementationResearchFindings/fs/en [accessed 16/8/05].
3 Griffiths F, Green E and Tsouroufli M (2005) The nature of medical evidence and its inherent uncertainty for the clinical consultation: qualitative study. *BMJ*. **330**: 511.
4 Boutron I, Ravaud P and Giraudeau B (2005) Inappropriateness of randomised trials for complex phenomena: single trial is never enough evidence to base decisions on. *BMJ*. **330**: 94.
5 Druss B (2005) Evidence based medicine: does it make a difference? Use wisely. *BMJ*. **330**: 92.
6 Ausubel DP (1960) The use of advance organizers in the learning and retention of meaningful verbal material. *Journal of Educational Psychology*. **51**: 267–72.
7 Honey P (2005) Honey & Mumford Learning Styles Questionnaire. www.peterhoney. co.uk.
8 Ruby3 (2005) Honey & Mumford's Learning Styles [An excellent introduction, simple to use – you should access this in conjunction with www.peterhoney.co.uk] www. ruby3.dircon.co.uk/Training%20Files/Theory%20Pages/learning%20styles.htm [accessed 9/6/06].
9 Kolb DA (1984) *Experiential Learning: experience as the source of learning and development*. Prentice-Hall, Englewood Cliffs, NJ.
10 Wilkinson A, Forbes A, Bloomfield J and Fincham GC (2004) An exploration of four web-based open and flexible learning modules in post-registration nurse education. *International Journal of Nursing Studies*. **41**: 411–24.
11 Waters M, Mohanna K and Deigton M (2002) Teaching Resources for Trainers. www.trainer.org.uk/resources.htm [accessed 27/9/02].
12 Quirck ME (1994) Recognizing and reducing the impact of individual learning differences. In: ME Quirck (ed.) *How To Learn and Teach in Medical School: a learner-centred approach*. Charles C Thomas: Springfield, IL.
13 Vygotsky LS (1978) *Mind in Society*. Cambridge University Press, Cambridge, MA.

Chapter 6

Blended learning

Gary Motteram

Key points

- Most educators have materials that they can make use of straight away.
- Finding the right blend depends on the learners and not the technology.
- There are many technologies but always keep it simple.
- Blended learning is an effective and efficient first step when starting with e-learning.

Introduction

Blended learning is a term that has been used in recent years to describe activities in learning that in the past have been called flexible learning. The idea of blending learning activities is not particularly new but is attracting more attention because a blended approach seems to be an efficient and effective way forward for many institutions wanting to make better use of information and communication technology (ICT) and e-learning. Most educators will have their learning materials in some kind of electronic (digital) format, even if these are only Word files or the occasional PowerPoint slide. However, many also have other digital materials, such as high quality pictures, video or audio clips, and links to useful websites and pages as educational resources. Blending, as its names implies, is a process in which digital resources can be mixed with the range of techniques that are already being used in teaching, such as lectures and seminars, group work or problem-based learning sessions. Educators are usually already familiar and confident with these techniques. The idea of blended learning is to combine the different elements of digital material with existing techniques so that optimum learning opportunities can be provided for learners. The educator needs to ask: how can the technology be used most effectively?[1]

What to consider when choosing how best to deliver digital material

The central issue is the learner, as with all curriculum development, and in our case adult learners. Adult learners come to the learning context with a considerable background in learning, some successful, some less successful; they also have certain propensities towards ways of learning, often called learning styles (audio/video/kinaesthetic); they may come equipped with a range of strategies that have been helpful to them in the past and they may have certain ideas about how they learn best. The younger they are, the more likely they are to have experienced learning using technology.

Important considerations for the educator are the range and ease of access to the technology, the cost to set it up and maintain it, and how much time it is going to take to develop. A first consideration might be to build on what is already in the environment, rather than trying something new that would take a lot of time and use up too much resource. Starting in too complicated a fashion may result in the project not succeeding, with the consequence that both the learner and educator are put off trying to do it again!

Selecting the right blend

It is not a good idea to start by looking at the technology. The use of Bates's[2] acronym (ACTIONS) is very useful as a general guide:

- **Access:** This is concerned with how easy it is for learners to utilise the materials. How technical is the material? Does it require specialist equipment to work? Do they have to travel to use it, or can they get it from home, or work? Do they need specialist training?
- **Costs:** These are both the costs of development and the costs to the end user. Is it cost-effective to create and deliver? Does it represent value for money? If the students are already paying a lot for a course, does this add to their outlay?
- **Teaching and learning:** Does it effectively fit with current ideas about teaching and learning? Is it going to enhance teaching and learning strategy?
- **Interactivity and user-friendliness:** Does the material have interactive elements which enhance the learning experience e.g. a glossary, high quality video clips that show how things work, links to searchable databases etc? Is it easy to use? Is it clear and well-designed?
- **Organisational issues:** How well does the use of this material fit in with current organisational policy? Does the organisation have the technologies available that we want to use? Is there local funding available to help in the development? How much support can be expected from the organisation or department? Are there other people doing similar things who can act as collaborators?
- **Novelty:** Sometimes there may be a desire to try an approach that is not a stable technology, but perhaps it is impressive. The reason may be that the developer is the first in their field to use it and the course can be made to seem up-to-date and ground-breaking. Sometimes it's better to start with a technology that is stable and well accepted to build the confidence of the developer.
- **Speed:** How long is it going to take to do what is planned? Is it easy to make changes and to update material once it has been produced? Sometimes relying on others to help can slow the process down.

Box 6.1 The range of possible technologies

- web-based courseware
- CD-ROM-based courseware
- live virtual classrooms

- web seminars
- conference calls
- virtual labs
- simulations
- online electronic resources
- portals

Starting with simple ideas first

The most obvious starting point is when there is a desire to increase the access to existing courses or when there is a need to provide supplementary learning materials to add value to a course.

What many tutors do as a starting point is to put lecture notes and PowerPoint slides online. This is often derided as an easy way out, but this approach can have a number of advantages, particularly if the educator can only slowly add to the resource. The lecture notes can be enhanced so that they become more comprehensive, or an audio track can be added to the PowerPoint slides to make this an online lecture. This may help learners to prepare in advance for a topic and the face-to-face meeting can be used for discussion. There is also the advantage that if learners are unable to attend a session; they have an online resource and extra copies of handouts do not have to be made available. As time goes by, embedded links can be added into the materials that are directed to other useful resources on the web, including direct links to a library database of articles that sits on the web. If learners are already expected to do some pre-course reading, then these can also be placed on the web so that they can be looked up in advance. These documents do not need to be produced as complex HTML files (files made ready to go on the web) but can be simple Word files that are uploaded on the website and which the user can easily access. Once a growing collection of learning materials begins to develop, it requires systematic organisation so that it does not appear cluttered and the learning materials are appropriately linked together.

If the learners are distributed in various places, they can be brought together to conduct online seminars. A simple email distribution list can warn the learners that they need to look at the task that has been set on the web. This task is linked to a set of articles, or scenarios, or case studies. They can discuss this material and come up with a solution. This seminar can be text-based, such as in a discussion board, by a live audio chat room or by the use of desk-top video conferencing using web-cams.

Conclusions

Getting started with e-learning is not that difficult, particularly if a blended approach is used. It is always a good idea to start from what the educator knows works well and what is already available in previous face-to-face sessions. It is important not to begin by selecting a particular technology but to choose the technology that will maximise the learning opportunity.

References

1 Bersin J (Undated) What works in blended learning. ASTD's Source for e-learning www.learningcircuits.org/2003/jul2003/bersin.htm [accessed 3 September 2005].
2 Bates AW (1995) *Technology, Open Learning and Distance Education*. Routledge, London.

Chapter 7

Collaborative knowledge sharing: an e-learning approach

John Sandars

Key points

- Collaborative sharing of professional knowledge is an important aspect of education for healthcare professionals.
- Exciting opportunities for communication are possible using the latest technology.
- 'Blogs' and 'wikis' offer novel approaches to informal knowledge sharing.
- Effective online collaborative learning requires structure and facilitation.

Introduction

The joining together of individuals to share knowledge and experiences has been recognised as an essential part of professional education for many years. However, most professionals are busy people, with the result that there are limited opportunities to meet face-to-face. In addition, many professionals are widely geographically dispersed. Despite these difficulties, there is an increasing need to share professional knowledge in the present complex world of healthcare. The growth of information and communications technology (ICT) can provide new possibilities.

Taking collaborative learning online

Effective collaborative learning requires individuals to participate, contribute and to have ownership of the learning. This process can be helped by appropriate ICT but the key factors that facilitate successful collaborative learning must be remembered. The development of trust and shared understanding is complex, requiring a mix of verbal and non-verbal communication. However, the online environment can amplify any possible difficulties. Online communication is usually dependent on the written word, with the consequence that there is a lack of crucial non-verbal cues that are essential for building trust and showing that communication is understood. Despite these difficulties, research has demonstrated that if these factors are considered in the development process for an online communication approach then effective collaborative learning can occur.[1]

Over the last few years there have been rapid developments in a variety of 'social software' products to help individuals communicate by an electronic method. Clay Shirky has defined social software as 'software that supports group interaction'.[2]

- **Instant messaging:** Instant messaging allows immediate one-to-one communication with other people. Colleagues can be added to a contact list and, if they are online, their name will be listed as available for chat. Clicking on their name will activate a chat window which has space to write to the other person and this also allows replies to be read. Popular applications include Yahoo Messenger, MSN Messenger and AOL Instant Messenger.
- **Internet Relay Chat (IRC):** allows users to join a chat room and communicate with many people at once. Users may join a pre-existing chat room or create a chat room about any topic. Once inside, messages from everyone else in the room can be read and replies can be sent to either a specific person or to all users. Usually there is a steady stream of people entering and leaving. A popular application is Yahoo Chat, which has a large variety of chat rooms.
- **Internet forums:** These allow users to post a topic for others to review, similar to a bulletin board. Other users can view the topic and post their own comments in a linear fashion, one after the other, to form a 'thread'. Most forums will require registration and there is control of the membership. Examples can be found at BMJ Learning and Doctors.net.uk.
- **Blogs or weblogs:** Blogs, short for web logs, are like online journals for a particular person. The owner posts a message and sometimes there is the opportunity for others to add their own comments. Topics often include the owner's daily life or views on a particular subject important to them. Examples include the BMJ Blogs in BMJ Careers.
- **Wikis:** A wiki is like a web page that allows users to add content, as on an internet forum, but they also allow anyone to edit the content. The main advantage of a wiki is the ease with which pages can be created and updated. Most wikis are open to the general public and do not require registration. Examples include Wikipedia and Wiktionary.
- **Virtual worlds and Massively-Multiplayer Online Games (MMOGs):** Virtual worlds and Massively-Multiplayer Online Games are places where it is possible to meet and interact with other people in a virtual world. Non-commercial, open-source and experimental examples include VOS and Solipsis. These approaches tend to be limited to those individuals who are very technically minded.

Additional approaches to increase collaborative learning

The usefulness of the main methods can be increased by newer approaches. These include notification when new messages have been posted, the ability to communicate by media other than text, accessibility from a variety of mobile devices and the opportunity to actively search for other people to communicate with.

- **Notification of new messages:** RSS (Real Simple Syndication) searches across multiple websites, such as blogs and wikis, to identify when new messages have been posted that are relevant to the particular needs of an individual. The person can be immediately notified and messages can be easily transmitted to a mobile phone.

- **Range of communication media:** Originally the main method of electronic communication was by passing text messages but the latest technology allows visual and auditory messages to be used.
- **Use of mobile devices:** The latest 3G mobile phones, especially those with personal digital assistant (PDA) functionality, allow ease of access to websites. This creates the opportunity for mobile phones to act as a remote interface with blogs and wikis.
- **Social network services:** Social network services allow people to come together online around shared interests. This type of sophisticated software also allows users to share blogs and instant messages. An existing example is the approach by online dating services where users can post their personal profiles and are able to search for a partner. This approach is being developed to link anyone with specific interests.

Getting started

The most important first step is to consider what can be expected from the use of an electronic method to facilitate communication. It is also essential to remember that communicating by a method that predominantly relies on written text requires a particular approach that some people may find difficult when it comes to adequately expressing their views.

Instant messaging, chat rooms and internet forums provide an ideal way to engage in a virtual conversation about a topic, although the method will be restricted by the amount of text within the messages that are exchanged. Most people dislike reading through large amounts of text without any visual enhancement.

Blogs and wikis present users with a website that has visual appeal and they also allow images to be posted. It is very easy to develop and launch an individual blog or wiki. No specialist knowledge of computer technology is required and within minutes anyone can have a presence on the World Wide Web. It is easy to restrict access by the use of passwords. Free publicly available software includes Blogger (www.blogger.com/) and Jotspot (www.jot.com/).

Online moderation

The online communication may be moderated, in which an online facilitator works with the participants, or unmoderated. Research suggests that learners in healthcare prefer structure to their online communication,[3] but online facilitation requires specific skills. Gilly Salmon offers a widely adopted approach that uses specific skills in a step-wise way to facilitate (also called 'e-moderation') online discussions: there is initial socialisation, followed by structured tasks and finally ongoing more distant support that allows autonomous learning.[4]

'Blogs' and 'wikis' for informal knowledge sharing

Most of the collaborative approaches have developed from organisations that have traditionally provided educational opportunities, such as higher education institutions or professional organisations. In response to the perceived control over the content that is discussed within these organisational contexts, there has recently been increasing interest in the use of 'blogs' and 'wikis'.[5] There is no shortage of existing blogs to choose from. Technorati (www.technorati.com) currently offers links to over 15.4 million blogs worldwide! Some are relevant to healthcare professionals, such as Family Medicine Notes (www.docnotes.com) or Medpundit (www.medpundit.blogspot.com), but many reflect the wide variety of interests that individuals have, both weird and not so unusual. This approach to knowledge sharing encourages rapid responses by readers, with almost immediate updating of the website. The websites are very idiosyncratic, reflecting the particular interests of the author, and this is the dilemma. Undoubtedly this is informal learning at the extreme – there is no control over the content and access is very easy. The reader has to carefully evaluate what they are reading.

Conclusion

Online opportunities to share professional knowledge offer an exciting future approach to e-learning in GP education. However, the experiences outlined in Chapters 2, 15 and 16 show that there is often poor engagement and the level of knowledge sharing is superficial. The technology to support online collaborative learning is available now but it needs acceptance by potential users, combined with adaptation to the different method of communication that the technology requires.

References

1 Hildreth PM, Kimble C and Wright P (2000) Communities of practice in the distributed international environment. *Journal of Knowledge Management.* **4**(1): 27–37.
2 Shirsky C (2003) A group is it's own worst enemy. http://shirky.com/writings/group_enemy.html.
3 Fox NJ, Dolman EA, Lane P *et al.* (1999) The WISDOM project: training primary care professionals in informatics in a collaborative 'virtual classroom'. *Medical Education.* **33**: 365–70.
4 Salmon G (2000) *E-moderating: the key to teaching and learning on-line.* Kogan Page, London.
5 Treese W (2004) Putting it together: Open systems for collaboration. *netWorker.* **8**: 13–16.

Chapter 8

Choosing an e-learning product

John Sandars and Kieran Walsh

Key points

- There are a wide range of e-learning products, with variable quality.
- No uniform system of educational accreditation exists.
- It is important to evaluate the approach to both technology and learning.
- The choice often depends on individual preference.

Introduction

There is an ever-increasing range of e-learning products and it is essential for all consumers to make an appropriate choice. This will help to reduce the frustration, and often the financial cost, of making a choice that is unsuitable.

e-learning can provide an excellent learning experience. High quality multimedia presentations can effectively convey difficult concepts and there may be the opportunity to communicate with a range of colleagues, including those overseas. This experience can be at a time and place convenient to the learner. However, this experience can be the opposite!

Developments in e-learning have often been dominated by technology, with the result that consideration of the educational process has sometimes been of secondary importance for e-learning product developers. There is a range of delivery systems using a variety of methods, such as CD-ROMs or web-based courses. This can offer a useful range of options for using the material. It is also important to consider not only how the educational content is being delivered but why it is being delivered in that format. These considerations maybe related to cost or the convenience to produce rather than responding to the needs of the consumer.

The key questions to consider

There are three useful screening questions to consider when choosing any e-learning product.

Is the learner ready to become an e-learner?

Becoming an e-learner requires a different approach to learning. This is in addition to using the technology.

Most e-learning will be a solitary experience, with little direct and immediate interaction with fellow learners. This requires a certain amount of self-discipline. It is also surprising that some potential e-learners do not appreciate that e-learning is delivered by computer-based technology! Most e-learning does not require anything more than simple keyboard skills but some people do appear to have a 'computerphobia'.

It is important to consider where and how the e-learning is going to be used. Often there will be the need to have access to a computer and sometimes the internet. Consideration has to be given to where e-learning will take place – home or place of work. Often at home there are conflicting domestic pressures on both time and access to the technology.

Is the provider well known as an e-learning provider?

Undoubtedly, previous personal experience of a provider can be very useful but there can be no guarantee! Often there is loyalty to a particular educational provider, such as a professional body.

Is the e-learning product, or provider, accredited by anyone?

Accreditation of e-learning is a complex area at the present time. There is no uniform or national system. Sometimes the e-learning product alone, and sometimes the e-learning provider alone form the basis for accreditation. Accreditation can provided by various Royal Colleges, such as the Royal College of Physicians or the Royal College of General Practitioners.

Evaluating the technology

The two main factors are the technical requirements, including access, and whether the technology is used appropriately.

Technical requirements

- **What equipment is required?** It is essential to be aware of the exact technical requirements to use the e-learning product. For example, there may be minimum levels of computer power or memory.
- **Is internet access required, especially broadband?** Many web-based e-learning products have been developed for use by university students or learners within large organisations. These groups usually have ready access to fast downloads and do not pay for the time whilst online. e-learning products that have a large proportion of highly visual material or are multimedia maybe very slow to download without broadband.
- **Is the 'platform stable'?** This jargon refers to how often the system 'goes down'.
- **What technical support is available?** There is always the possibility that the technology can fail and it is essential to have good technical support. This may require a service that can be used 24 hours every day, including Bank Holidays. It really depends on the expected time that the learner will be studying.

Appropriate use of technology

- **Is it easy to navigate?** This jargon refers to how easy it is to move around the e-learning product. For example, moving between materials may require constant return to the introductory page rather then a click on the page.
- **Is the use of multimedia designed to enhance learning or does it distract the user?**
- **Are key messages reinforced by different methods, such as by a combination of text, visual and auditory forms?**
- **Are any links to the internet live, and if so, are they regularly checked?** Many e-learning products link to useful websites and it is helpful if these links can be activated without moving out of the product.

Evaluating the educational approach

What does the product cost?

- Is it free or is there a charge to access?
- How often is access provided after any payment?

Many high quality e-learning products are freely available on the internet but it is not always obvious, if payment is required, whether it is 'one-off' or whether it can be accessed several times over a period of time.

What is the learning content?

- Is it clearly described?
- Is it up to date? When was it last updated?
- Is it relevant to the learning needs of the learner?
- Is it peer-reviewed?
- Is it written by GPs or hospital doctors?
- Is it written for GPs or hospital doctors?
- Can the materials be studied with other healthcare professionals, such as with the practice nurse or practice manager?

It is easy to get a preview of the learning content of a book by simply turning over the pages. However, it is often difficult to see the content for many e-learning products without initial payment or registration for an access password.

How are the learning materials presented?

- Is it in the form of an interactive case history?
- Is it in the form of lecture notes or textbooks?

Most people learn best by an active process rather than by reading through large amounts of text. Technology has the power to store large amounts of factual information within a small amount of space, but it can also offer superb opportunities to provide interactive quizzes that aid more effective learning.

What is the learning process?

- How much time is the learner expected to spend on the learning?
- Is the learner actively engaged with the learning materials, such as interacting with the media or being prompted to find out further information?
- Is learning linked to real-life situations?
- Is there any feedback on the learning, such as through a quiz?

What will the learner obtain at the end of the period of learning?

- What is the learner expected to have learnt?
- Will any credits, certificates or academic award be given?
- Is there a system for keeping a log of the learning that has been done?

A recent trend in e-learning is the development of learning management systems that allow learners to identify their learning needs, make choices of what they wish to learn and then keep a record of what has been learnt. This allows the development of an 'e-portfolio'.

Is there an opportunity to communicate with other learners?

- What method is available?
- Is it by email or by the use of a discussion board?
- Is this process facilitated by a tutor or mentor? This is called 'moderated discussion'.

Most learners appreciate the opportunity to share experiences with other learners, and this is an important part of any learning experience. Technology can help this process by developing communication channels between learners, either informally or formally. It is possible to establish a good group discussion between learners, sometimes facilitated by a tutor, but it requires getting used to the barriers imposed by the technology, such as relying on a communication by text and not being able to reply and read messages at the same time.

Do the learning providers provide evidence that they are operating to high ethical standards?

- Will the use of the website be completely confidential (that is, will only the user be able to know what learning modules that they have completed)?
- Do the providers declare any conflicts of interest?

Many e-learning providers have strong sponsorship, either from pharmaceutical companies or from a wide variety of commercial and personal service providers, such as office supplies.

Conclusion

e-learning products can offer an effective and high quality learning experience but, like all purchases, the consumer has to be aware! There is no ideal product but a critical evaluation should allow the learner to make an informed choice.

Chapter 9

Standards and accreditation for e-learning

Zoe Barker

Key points

- Accreditation evaluates providers against established standards to ensure a high level of educational quality.
- Several systems for accreditation currently exist, each with different criteria.
- There are inequalities in accreditation between web-based and computer-based e-learning.
- UK general practice is leading the way on the accreditation of online learning.

Introduction

The accreditation of online learning is a validation process by which education providers are evaluated against established standards to ensure a high level of educational quality.[1] To provide accredited courses, and to be an accredited education provider of online continuing medical education (CME), the provider must meet a set of stringent standards and criteria. This chapter highlights the range of different approaches for accreditation of e-learning.

EACCME: European Accreditation Council for CME

In an ever-increasing global market it is clear that there is a need for a visible quality system, with standard definitions and control to realise global harmonisation. Since CME systems evolve independently in each European state, doctors attending events outside of their home country would experience problems in collecting 'valid' CME credits.

The European Accreditation Council for CME (EACCME) was established in January 2000, to act as a clearing house system for international CME accreditation. Its purpose is to facilitate the international transfer and recognition of CME credits obtained by individuals in CME activities that meet common quality requirements.[2]

EACCME aims to connect existing and emerging accreditation systems:

- between European countries
- between different specialties
- in case of migration of specialists within Europe
- between the European accreditation system and comparable systems outside Europe.

The EACCME establishes standards and procedure that need to be applied by the accrediting authorities. EACCME delegates the task of review and accreditation to Boards within medical specialties such as the European Board for Accreditation of Cardiology (EBAC).

The accreditation criteria for the EACCME are:

- **Integral learner support:** The learner is provided with an introduction to the course, to include at least the following:
  - the purpose of the course
  - learning objectives
  - the structure of the course
  - estimated required study time
  - estimated elapsed time required to complete the course
  - any materials (books, software etc.) to be supplied by the learner
  - the hardware and software required to use the materials
  - how to get the best from the course.

The learner is provided with instructions on using the course, to include at least the following:

- **Content:**
  - Given the support of online tutors, where provided, is sufficient to allow the learner to reach the learning objectives.
  - Structured into meaningful sections and arranged into a sequence and/or hierarchy that facilitates learning.
  - Written at a level appropriate to the specified audience.
  - Lively, stimulating and enjoyable.
  - Free of intended or unintended racist, sexist or ageist material.
  - Accurate, up-to-date and free of spelling and grammatical errors.
  - Does not violate existing copyrights.
  - All units include an overview and summary.
- **Learning design:** Uses a variety of approaches designed to satisfy the needs of learners with different learning styles. Adequate provision is made in the design for the learner to:
  - reflect on, review and digest new learning
  - apply new knowledge and practise new skills
  - assess their progress.
- **Methods and media are selected appropriately** according to their suitability in helping the learner to achieve the particular learning objective.
- **Opportunities for meaningful user interaction** are provided regularly throughout the course, whether built into the materials or through communication with other learners and tutors.

  Where interactivity is built into the materials, questions are set at a level appropriate to the audience.
- **Pre- and post-assessment:** Sufficient tests, exercises or assignments are

included to ensure the learner has achieved all of the learning objectives. Where appropriate, the materials include an optional facility for pre-assessment of the learner's existing knowledge, skills or attitudes. Where pre- or post-assessments are employed, it is clear where results are stored and how they will be used.

Buttons are provided to allow the learner to exit the current section, move upwards within a hierarchy of menus and, from the top level, to exit.

- **Usability:** The course conforms to best practice with regard to readability: text is legible against the background and appropriate fonts are selected.
- **Media quality:** At the specified minimum bandwidth, the time taken to load any image, animation, applet, movie, sound file or document is acceptable given the instructional purpose. The delay should not be greater than 10 seconds.
  - Audio is free from unnecessary hiss, page turns, lip smacks and other extraneous noise and is not clipped at the front or the end.
- **Technical quality:** The program is free of software bugs and broken links.
  - Images display intelligibly at the minimum supported colour resolution.
  - Where delivered as a web application, the program runs without error on all supported brands and versions of browsers and browser add-ons such as plug-ins.
  - The program runs without error on all supported types of computer, at the minimum supported specification.

Primary Care CPD (PDP & PPDP) accreditation

On 1 April 2004, the Postgraduate Education Allowance (PGEA) was included into the global sum of the new General Medical Services contract.[3] PGEA was replaced by Continuing Professional Development (CPD) because it did not consistently deliver high quality continuing medical education leading to an improvement in patient care. CPD consists of Personal Development Plans (PDP) and Practice Development Plans (PPDP). PDPs are aimed at managing doctors' education and professional development and PPDP at managing the practice's organisational development. Together, PDP and PPDP aim to bridge the gap between time spent on learning and application of what was learnt. CPD combines documented personal learning within an organisational development framework.[4]

In terms of the accreditation criteria for an educational resource, very little has changed in the switch from PGEA to CPD. Accreditation is by the UK Council of Educational Advisors and administered via a distance-based learning panel c/o the Royal College of General Practitioners.

The CPD accreditation criteria are detailed as follows.

- **Relevance to general practice:** The topics must be in an area likely to address a clearly identified educational need in general practice or to general practitioners.
- **Quality of course materials:** Material supplied should be of good written quality, with adequate audio-visual/computer-assisted learning material where appropriate. The package should be clearly laid out and easily navigable by participants.

- **Clarity of educational aims and objectives:** Aims and objectives should be clear and include identifiable learning outcomes.
- **Degree of interaction:** Packages should encourage interaction with tutors, other participants, or through personalised feedback to individual participants.
- **Assessment of performance:** Packages should include sufficient elements of objective evaluation to ensure that educational benefit is derived from it.
- **Amount of reflection:** Packages should specifically aim to encourage reflection through the use of personal case material, individual workplace scenarios, individual contact and/or feedback and interaction between participants. Material should encourage participants to change their clinical practice or organisation.
- **Feedback from learners:** Programmes should include an evaluation of the effectiveness of the programme by learners, which is used to modify and improve the programme on an ongoing basis.

The package/course/activity must meet the following criteria:

- Involve a GP tutor and/or a GP educationalist in its planning; should where possible encourage needs-based learning with an emphasis towards encouraging reflective and/or team-based learning; the educational content of the programme should be decided by a named educational adviser. The educational experience of the adviser should be included in the application. Programme providers should be asked to identify the interactive component of the programme including all methods of interaction and all persons who are involved in interacting with course participants.
- Packages/programmes must contain no promotional activity as an integral part of the programme. All applications must include any accompanying material mailed out with the educational programme or relating to it.
- From April 2004 materials/topics need not relate to any of the three following PGEA subject areas although providers will be asked to provide information about the broad area covered by the programme:
  - Subject Area One: Health Promotion
  - Subject Area Two: Disease Management
  - Subject Area Three: Service Management.
- Programme providers should identify an independent person who will evaluate the programme and submit a report under the headings above, including suggestions for modification.
- At the end of the activity, the UK National Accreditation Panel will require an Annual Report.

HPD accreditation

As well as clinical issues, doctors must meet educational objectives in areas such as practice organisation and management, team working, audit and research. Higher professional development (HPD) would allow areas such as practice organisations, audit and research, which cannot always be considered in depth during the single year in practice in Vocational Training. Higher professional education would be done on a voluntary basis, for a minimum period of two years. There would be no maximum time limit and the total length of time should be determined by the educational needs of the doctor.[4]

HPD accreditation criteria includes:

1 **Course/materials rationale:** The course/materials should derive from an assessment of unmet need or demand from general practice/primary care. The rationale for the mode of delivery (i.e. distance-, tutor-based, research-based etc.) should be clear and convincing.

2 **Aims/objectives:** There must be a clear description of the educational aims and objectives of the course or learning materials so that participants are aware of the learning which they can be expected to experience and how learning outcomes can be measured. The aims and objectives and learning outcomes should be appropriate to general practitioners. They should be clear to learners and reflected in the content, design and delivery of the course/materials. There should be an indication of the time needed for taught elements and private study.

3 **Relation to Good Medical Practice (GMP) and Good Medical Practice for General Practice:** All RCGP-accredited courses and learning materials must be mapped onto the relevant sections of GMP. The linkages with GMP need to be demonstrated so that GPs undertaking the course or programme of learning can use evidence from this process for their appraisal and revalidation folders. Linkage into Good Medical Practice for GPs is desirable. These linkages will also enable participants on the College's Accredited Professional Development Programme to see how the course or materials can be used to fulfil its requirements.

4 **Selection/admission process and criteria (courses only):** These should ensure that GPs selected onto the course will be able to benefit from it e.g. understand what is involved; have the prerequisite knowledge, skills and experience. GPs should be aware of the advantages and disadvantages of particular delivery methods, including time commitment, so they can make an informed choice.

5 **Guidance on who will benefit from the materials (learning materials only):** The materials should indicate clearly and realistically what previous under-standing or experience is needed to benefit from them, how much time will be required to work through them and what software and other support is needed.

6 **Access and equal opportunities (courses):** The course should allow for the whole range of GPs who might benefit from access to the course. There should be an equal opportunities policy, covering access, delivery and assessment, and evidence of how it is operated.

7 **Equal opportunities and anti-discrimination (materials):** There should be policy stating how the materials are reviewed to ensure they contain no language or content which would cause offence.

8 **Course/materials design:** The rationale for the design of the course/learning. Materials and the underpinning model of teaching and learning should be described.

9 **Course/materials content:** There should be evidence that this is relevant to GPs. There should be a process for reviewing and updating the content, and for incorporating relevant national and professional body policy. The content should be coherent and manageable in the specified time. There should be no promotional material in the course and any sponsorship should be clearly stated.

10 **Relating the course to practice (courses only):** There should be mechanisms

for GPs to get feedback on their progress and for difficulties with progress be identified and supported. There should also be processes to relate learning to a personal and/or practice development plan. Please describe how you encourage the transfer of learning to practice and facilitate GPs integrating their own experience with the learning from the course. Tuition should encourage and facilitate a self-reflective and participative form of learning which will allow participants to review their needs during the course, although this doesn't exclude a didactic component.

11 **Support for learning (materials only):** There should be clear guidance on how to work through the materials to get greatest benefit from them. There should be built-in feedback mechanisms and encouragement to reflect on learning and relate it to practice. There should be access to help with technical difficulties. Opportunities for face-to-face or other forms of personal support are desirable.

12 **Monitoring and evaluation (materials only):** There should be evidence of mechanisms for obtaining and acting on feedback from users. There should be evidence of regular review of the materials.

Practice accreditation

The practice accreditation scheme was first developed and piloted by the Royal College of General Practitioners Scottish Council in 1999. It has been designed as a tool that will encourage and help all members of the practice-based primary care team to take the first step in meeting standardised quality criteria. The focus should be the team, its functioning and the services it provides. Assessment should be multidisciplinary and there should be local ownership and delivery.[5]

Quality Practice Award (QPA)

QPA is a quality assurance process undertaken by practices. It is awarded in recognition of a high standard of patient care delivered by every member of the primary care team.

Quality Team Development (QTD) (England only)

QTD aims to help primary care groups (PCGs) and primary care trusts (PCTs) assess the performance of primary care teams. Assessment methods include a practice self-assessment questionnaire, practice profile, patient questionnaires, documentation review and a practice visit by a team (usually a GP, nurse and practice manager) which undertakes direct observation, interviews and clinical record review.

Practice Accreditation (PracA) (Scotland only)

PracA covers a wide range of clinical and service criteria applicable to patients and to the primary care team. The 127 criteria are in three categories: Essential, Good and Quality. Practices must meet all 46 Essential criteria, and must demonstrate that they can also meet a maximum of a further 20 criteria, which should be a mixture of Good and Quality criteria, thus demonstrating that they have in place the essential elements to provide good general practice.

Primary Care Research Team Assessment (PCRTA)

PCRTA is an assessment process which focuses on primary care research teams within individual practices.

Two levels of assessment are available:

- **PCRTA Collaborator Research Practice:** Practices relatively new to research benefit from completing assessment at this level if they wish to move forward to undertaking higher quality research.
- **PCRTA Investigator-led Research Practice:** A practice having a significant track record of sound research, and evidence of it informing their practice and improving the health of the relevant local populations

EPASS (Scotland) accreditation

The Educational Providers Accreditation Scheme (Scotland) (EPASS) awards accreditation to education providers who want to gain recognition for their commitment to quality education. The scheme also provides assurance to general practitioners who want to know that any continuing professional development (CPD) activities they undertake are relevant to their needs. RCGP Scotland continues to work with NHS Education for Scotland to ensure that GP appraisers are aware of EPASS and the significance of an EPASS event within a doctor's appraisal folder.[6]

The details for EPASS quality criteria are set out in Box 9.1.

Box 9.1 EPASS quality criteria

Providers acknowledge and agree that the following conditions apply to all EPASS events.

- There must be a named individual responsible for each EPASS event whose identity is suitably clear to those attending the event and to EPASS.
- If the event provider is not a general practitioner then there must be access to a named general practitioner for advice during the EPASS event.
- Wherever possible, the provider should encourage needs-based learning with an emphasis towards reflective learning and a variety of learning based methods should be used during the EPASS event.
- Delegates at EPASS events must be provided with the opportunity for active participation in a learning activity and must receive feedback on their performance during the event, where appropriate.
- EPASS events must not contain any promotional activity as an integral part of the programme.
- Delegates attending EPASS events must be made aware that their contact

details may be passed to the EPASS Scrutiny Panel for the sole purpose of carrying out random assessment.
- EPASS events may be randomly assessed by questionnaire to delegates or by a formal review undertaken by the EPASS Scrutiny Panel.

Secondary Care Royal College accreditation

The Royal Colleges provide mutual accreditation for educational courses/activities. The Academy of Medical Royal Colleges (AOMRC) co-ordinates the work of the medical Royal Colleges and faculties, and specifies the 10 principles for Colleges' accreditation, which are:

1 College/Faculty CPD schemes should be available to all Members and Fellows and, at reasonable cost, to non-Members and Fellows who practise in a relevant specialty.
2 Normally, units of College/Faculty CPD should be based on hours of participation, and the minimum required should be an average of 50 per year. Credits for untimed activities such as writing should be agreed between College/Faculty directors of CPD.
3 College/Faculty CPD should include a balance of activities both within and outside the employing institution, as well as a component of active learning.
4 An individual's CPD activities should reflect and be relevant to their profile of professional practice and performance. This should include continuing education outside narrower specialty interests.
5 Participation in College/Faculty-based CPD should be acknowledged by a regular statement issued to participants based on annually submitted returns of accrued credits.
6 Colleges/faculties should fully audit a participant's activities on a random basis or whenever concerns about an individual's professional performance are raised. Such peer-based audit should verify that claimed activities have been undertaken and are appropriate. Participants will need to collect evidence to enable this process, normally using a structured portfolio cataloguing the different activities.
7 The proportion of participants involved in random audit each year should be of a size to give confidence that it is representative and will vary according to the number of participants in a given scheme.
8 Formal endorsement of educational activities for CPD by Colleges/faculties can continue but should be achieved with the minimum bureaucracy and with complete reciprocity between Colleges/faculties for all approved events. Self-accreditation of relevant activities and documented reflective learning should also be allowed and encouraged.
9 To enable self-accreditation of events, formal CPD certificates of attendance at meetings will not be a requirement. Other evidence of attendance is acceptable (e.g. registration receipt, name badge, list of delegates or programme). Signed registers are only necessary where there is no other available evidence of attendance (e.g. grand rounds).
10 Failure when challenged to produce sufficient evidence to support claimed

credits will result in an individual's annual statement being endorsed accordingly for the year involved and their subsequently being subject to annual audit. Suspected falsification of evidence for claimed credits may result in referral to the GMC/GDC.

Web-based learning vs computer-based learning

e-learning covers a wide set of applications and processes, such as web-based learning, computer-based learning, virtual classrooms and online collaboration. Web-based learning includes online courses or any kind of educational resource that is on the World Wide Web, such as online classrooms or forums. Computer-based learning mainly encompasses offline learning through the use of computers or computer-based technology, such as an interactive CD-ROM.

Not all colleges accredit online courses, although these enable greater ability to audit and check than lunchtime lectures or seminars. For example, the Royal College of Physicians will accredit a course if it is on CD, but not if the same course is online. The EACCME does not accredit online courses either.

The accreditation criteria for a resource (e.g. a CD course) are as follows.

1 The target audience falls within the remit of the Federation (given medical specialties).
2 The content is concerned with clinical specialty-based issues or with the development of non-clinical skills (e.g. management, teaching, information technology etc.) necessary to work in a modern health service.
3 The package provides educational objectives for the user and a method of assessment to measure whether these objectives have been reached.
4 The package provides evidence of interactivity between the user and material to enhance the learning process.
5 The package is flexible and free from unreasonable geographical and resource (hardware and software) implications and time constraints that will restrict access to use.
6 Any sponsorship or funding has not influenced the educational programme content, and programme authors are completely independent of any commercial healthcare organisation.
7 The provider's evaluation record for previous events is satisfactory or, where not, reasons for unsatisfactory ratings have subsequently been addressed.
8 The provider agrees to submit, upon request, confirmation of physician participation at any time up to two years after the event has taken place.
9 Information and references should be relevant, up-to-date and where possible encompass the best evidence available, and it should also adequately cover the subject area without any inexplicable omissions appearance and functionality should be user-friendly.
10 There are appropriate methods of assessment included. Feedback for the user should be available in order to improve performance the final assessment and pass rate should be of a standard that is beneficial for CPD purposes.
11 Information provided by the producer should include:
   – results of any market research for need of such materials amongst intended users

- details of any evaluative procedures before and during the package's developmental stage.
12 The package should be a cost-effective and innovative contribution to a physician's learning environment and the range of CPD activities available.

Institute of IT Training (IITT) accreditation

To be IITT-compliant, the education provider, learning materials and developer (the individual practitioner) levels will be assessed, and current best practice in these areas defined. The standards are reviewed on an annual basis to ensure continued currency and applicability.[7]

The standards cover four main areas:

1 **Code of practice for e-learning providers:** e-learning providers must adhere to the terms of this code of practice and continually demonstrate that they do so to be eligible for accreditation by the Institute. Through this, the Institute will maintain and monitor a register of approved providers of e-learning.

The following areas are included in the code of practice:
 - publicity and promotion
 - course information
 - learning materials standards
 - third-party standards
 - developer competencies
 - tutor competencies
 - external controls
 - complaints procedure.
2 **e-learning provider accreditation programme:** Institute accreditation requires rigorous assessment by expert practitioners and applicants commit to ongoing compliance with the Institute's code of practice.
3 **Standards for e-learning materials:** For e-learning to fulfil its promise, learning materials have to be designed so as to facilitate learning within a simulating whilst enjoyable environment. The standards focus on key areas:
 - integral learner support
 - content interactive design
 - navigation usability
 - media quality
 - technical quality.
4 **Competencies for developers of e-learning materials:** Best-practice competencies are evidence of which has to be shown by individual practitioners applying for membership of the Institute.

Further details on the accreditation scheme can be accessed at www.iitt.org.uk/

Conclusion

UK general practice is leading the way in the accreditation of online learning. The situation is less clear for both UK secondary care and healthcare across Europe.

DoctorOnline.nhs.uk is a major online medical course provider in the UK and is promoted by the NHS as the doctors' portal on the NHS Net. DoctorOnline.nhs.uk offers over 1000 hours of e-learning across the clinical spectrum.

References

1 elearners.com, Distance Learning Accreditation. www.elearners.com/resources/accreditation.asp.
2 European Board for Accreditation in Cardiology, EACCME, www.ebac-cme.org/newsite/archives/Vol%2001/eaccme1.pdf.
3 Life after PGEA (2004) *Pharmaceutical Field*. **6**: 14–15.
4 Royal College of General Practitioners, Higher Professional Development. www.rcgp.org.uk/education/higher_pro_dev.asp.
5 Royal College of General Practitioners – NI, Practice Accreditation. www.rcgp-ni.org.uk/ni/Practice%20Accreditation.htm.
6 Royal College of General Practitioners – Scotland, EPASS. www.rcgp-scotland.org.uk/development/epass.asp.
7 Institute of IT Training, Accreditation programme and code of practice for e-learning providers. www.iitt.org.uk/public/accreditation/elearn-prov.asp#Standards.

Chapter 10

The BMJ Learning approach to e-learning

Kieran Walsh

Key points

- BMJ Learning covers a broad range of topics (both clinical and non-clinical).
- It caters for the learning needs of practice nurses, practice managers and GP trainees as well as GPs.
- It provides learning resources to enable juniors to meet the needs of the new Foundation Year curriculum as set up by Modernising Medical Careers.
- Assessment of learning needs is linked to a personal and professional development.
- There are different types of learning resources on the site: interactive case histories, just in time modules and read, reflect, respond modules.
- Rapid responses allow users to contribute their ideas and share comments and learn from each other.
- Good content is essential. Learners are less concerned with how clever a website is and more concerned with whether they will learn anything useful from it.

Introduction

In 1995 Bates said that 'newer technologies such as computers and video conferencing are not necessarily better (or worse) for teaching or learning than older technologies . . . they are just different . . . the choice of technology should be driven by the needs of the learners and the context in which we are working, not by its novelty.'[1]

Ten years later we have a growing number of e-learning resources for general practitioners. BMJ Learning is just one of those resources. Is there any reason to think that is special? Is it truly driven by the needs of learners? Certainly it covers a broad range of topics (both clinical and non-clinical), it enables you to link your needs assessments with your personal and professional development plan and then with learning resources and so does live up to its name in that regard as 'a one-stop shop for e-learning'. It is also strongly evidence-based and takes its evidence from *Clinical Evidence* – a compendium of evidence-based practice in the

UK.[2] Its content is also updated every year and finally it has a lot of feedback which is published on the live site and which enables the learners and teachers to see what everyone's learning needs are and thus allows us – the editors – to try to meet those needs.

The BMJ Learning approach

In 2004 the BMJ launched BMJ Learning as an online resource to help GPs with their appraisal and revalidation. The idea was that if you have access to learning resources based on the best available evidence then you will be able to improve the quality of care that you provide to patients. If you can record your learning systematically then you will feel more confident about your appraisals and subsequent revalidation.

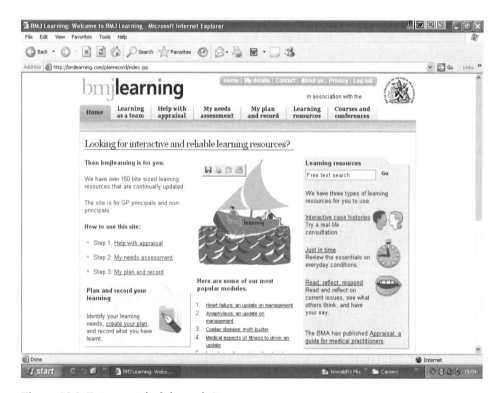

Figure 10.1 Entry portal of the website

BMJ Learning offers comprehensive support for your learning. It enables you to:

- find out about appraisal and revalidation
- assess your learning needs
- plan and record your learning
- do evidenced-based learning modules that are linked to the General Medical Services (GMS) contract, National Service Frameworks and NICE guidelines
- find out about courses and conferences near you with the courses and conferences guide.

It joins together all these features in a seamless way: you can link your learning needs with your learning plan and with the learning modules. The appraisal section of the website takes you through appraisal in a simple step-by-step fashion. It explains what an appraisal is and what you should expect from it. By now most doctors have passed through the process at least once and thus understand it. But if you are unsure and want to know what's involved and what your responsibilities are and what you should be getting out of it, then the appraisal pages are for you.

The learning needs assessment tools on the site enable you to find out what you need to know. There are a variety of methods of learning needs assessment to help you uncover the gaps in your knowledge, and different tools will suit different people. We debated about which ones to put on the site and decided to be quite catholic in our tastes and describe six of these tools. Examples of the tools include our PUNs and DENs (Patients' Unmet Needs and Doctors' Educational Needs) tools or our self-assessment tools or our 360-degrees appraisal tools.

The personal and professional development plan helps you to plan and record your learning. You can use the plan and record pages on this site to plan out the learning you are going to do over the next few weeks and months. You can then track your progress in fulfilling your plan.

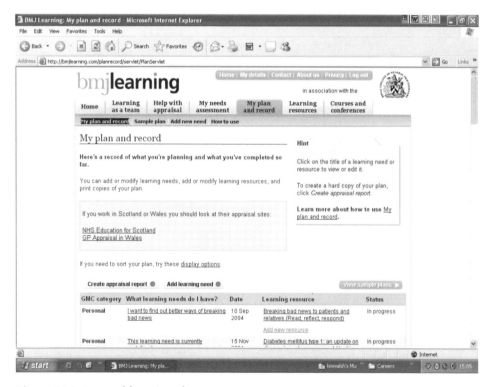

Figure 10.2 Personal learning plan

We strongly believe in the effectiveness of e-learning but we are not yet messianic in our beliefs. We realise that doctors don't want to do all their learning online and indeed we wouldn't encourage this. For this reason our growing database of conferences, seminars, lectures and workshops will help you find the meeting you need. You can search meetings by specialty, cost, childcare facilities and even by distance from your home. Because we update the database constantly you can be sure you won't miss any important activities. The idea is that no course or meeting will be too small to put in. And you can let us know about courses that you are running and we will put them up on the site. Currently we have over 200 courses and conferences on the site.

But the main wealth of the site is the learning modules. There are different types of learning resources on the site:

- interactive case histories enable you to train and test your consultation skills
- just-in-time modules offer bite-sized chunks of information
- read, reflect, respond modules allow you to read about a topic, think over the issues outlined, and give your opinions.

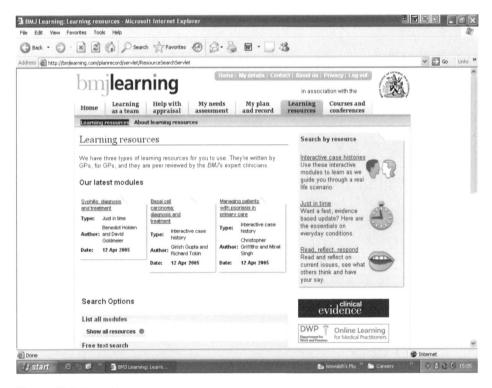

Figure 10.3 Learning resources

Throughout the learning modules we ask questions. We don't waste time testing trivial facts or asking tricky or unnecessarily complicated questions. Rather, we ask you questions on important aspects of a topic that require you to apply your knowledge. Our questions test your skills in interpreting data and making decisions, and they cover diagnosis, investigations, treatment and prognosis. You will receive immediate feedback on your answers. The learning modules are all evidenced-based and peer-reviewed and continually updated. They are built according to sound and modern educational principles. There are over 140 learning modules on the site. Where possible the learning modules are based on *Clinical Evidence*, clinical quality indicators in the new GMS contract, NICE guidelines and National Service Frameworks.

Box 10.1 The range of learning modules

Clinical areas:

- cardiology
- respiratory medicine
- gastroenterology
- endocrinology
- haematology
- neurology
- psychiatry
- rheumatology
- pain management
- drug information
- dermatology
- infectious diseases
- palliative care
- elderly care
- urology
- sexual health
- paediatrics
- women's health.

Non-clinical topics:

- clinical epidemiology
- communication skills
- ethics and law
- management and IT skills
- public health.

General Medical Council:

- maintaining good medical practice
- relationships with patients
- working with colleagues
- teaching and training, appraising, and assessing
- probity
- health and performance of colleagues.

Since the launch of the site over 33 000 health professionals have registered. The vast majority of them are UK GPs but some are hospital doctors from within the UK. There are over 3000 international users from over 130 countries. About 14% of users return to the site every two weeks. At the end of the learning modules we encourage users to give feedback and we have received over 20 000 individual pieces of feedback since the site began.

Recent developments

In October 2004 we launched a new interdisciplinary website: the new BMJ Learning caters for the learning needs of practice nurses and practice managers in primary care as well as GPs. The section of the site for practice nurses offers them suitable learning needs assessment tools and help with their performance reviews. There are also over 25 modules specifically for practice nurses. The section of the site for practice managers enables them to plan and record their learning and also offers them similar number of learning modules that are tailored to their specific learning needs. But all users will be able to access all the learning modules on the site. You can use the site as an individual but we do know of many people who use it as a team so they can learn together. For example, you could use our modules on diabetes and hypothyroidism as a foundation for a half-day's teaching on endocrinology. We feel that learning together has many advantages. You can learn information from each other and, more importantly, you can share different insights and perspectives on clinical and ethical dilemmas.

A recent addition to the site is the new section for junior hospital doctors. It caters for all juniors but it is likely that those training to become general practitioners will find it particularly useful. It provides learning resources to enable juniors to meet the needs of the new Foundation Year curriculum as set up by Modernising Medical Careers.[4,5]

The curriculum establishes what juniors should learn about – they should all learn basic skills in generic topics such as time management and communication and also emergency medicine skills such as how to care for someone with chest pain or with an acute asthma attack. All these topics are now covered by BMJ Learning.

A very recent addition to the site is learning resources for hospital specialists. Senior hospital doctors who looked at BMJ Learning wanted something similar for themselves. We have provided learning content for this user group and have initially concentrated on non-clinical topics such as how to set up a course. But they also get clinical modules which have a broad range of appeal – on topics such as antibiotic-resistant patterns to *Helicobacter pylori* and how to prevent contrast nephropathy. We have been delighted to publish some modules in association with the journals *Heart* and *Gut*. But in keeping with the sharing philosophy of BMJ Learning, all users including the general practitioners will be able to do these modules if they so wish.

Future developments

However, like any other learning product there is room for improvement and there are some things that we could do better. For example, users can send responses to us about individual BMJ learning modules. For some modules they are expansive in their thoughts and ideas. Other users can see their responses and respond to them – this adds a great deal to each individual learning resource. But there is at present no facility whereby users can communicate directly with each other. So how best to overcome this? One way is to set up a learning forum. Users could come to the forum and share ideas about recent innovations in medical education. They could also ask each other questions on clinical and non-clinical dilemmas. No learning resource can answer all possible questions on a particular subject but it is quite likely that someone else out there will have been in their situation before and will be able to help and give advice. The downside of some fora is that they can quickly deteriorate into a whingeing session for health professionals. They can become dominated by a small number of users who scare off others. The challenge for the BMJ Learning forum will be to keep health professionals concentrating and posting on relevant topics and being constructive in their criticisms and suggestions.

Another suggestion for the site is that we should make the site more multi-media. We have certainly considered this but so far have been judicial in our approach to multimedia learning. Donald Clark, a leading authority in multi-media learning in the UK, once said: 'Early multimedia learning looked like a car that had been cobbled together from different scrap yards with components of different sizes, colours, models and ages. It was a mongrel beast.' He was referring to the early flood of learning websites that had loud music and loud colour and even loud text. Videos popped up all over the screen and animation was everywhere. The designers loved it but learners were bemused and distracted. In the end they learned little. So far on bmjlearning.com we have erred on the side of multimedia learning for a purpose. Text is still very useful – experienced readers can read at a rate of 300 words per minute or slower if they wish to: everyone can read at their own pace. You can also search text quickly and we can easily update it. But we are building more multimedia content on the site. We have recently published new modules on dermatology and have many requests from users for more of this material. Traditionally colour slides are used to support text but here the pictures are at the core of the module. We show pictures of patients with different types of skin lesions and then test and train your skills in diagnosing and managing these conditions.

And how do we evaluate the site? Before we launched we decided to strongly encourage all learners to tell us what they thought of the learning materials that we have provided. We have been surprised by the number of responses that we have received – over 20 000 at the last count. The responses have been very positive. Other users can see the evaluation of modules before they start them in the same way that users of Amazon.co.uk can see other readers' opinions before they decide to purchase. This has enabled us to effectively democratise the site. Anyone can see which are the most popular modules. The most popular and most recent modules also change all the time and we thus have a top 10 of popular learning resources that changes constantly over time.

Conclusion

The original aims of BMJ Learning was to help doctors with their learning and in the process we have learned an enormous amount ourselves. One interesting thing that we learned is that even though it is an appraisal website the most popular modules are interactive case histories which enable you to assess your knowledge. We have also been surprised and delighted to see that the most challenging modules are also the most popular and we suspect that this shows that there is a real appetite for e-learning and education more generally in primary care. Finally we have learnt that good content is still king. Learners are less concerned with how clever a website is and more concerned with whether they will learn anything useful from it. If you want to have a look, just click on www.bmjlearning.com and off you go. We very much welcome your thoughts and suggestions.

References

1 Bates AW (1995) *Technology, Open Learning and Distance Education*. Routledge, London.
2 www.clinicalevidence.com/ceweb/conditions/index.jsp.
3 General Medical Council (2003) *A Licence to Practise and Revalidation*. GMC, London. (Also available at www.revalidationuk.info).
4 Crockard A (2005) The foundation programme curriculum – Q&As. *BMJ Career Focus*. **330**(April): 148.
5 Duncan R and Downey P (2004) Foundation programmes in general practice. *BMJ Career Focus*. **328**(May): 193–94.

Chapter 11

The Doctors.net.uk model of e-learning

Sue Lacey Bryant and Tim Ringrose

Key points

- Doctors.net.uk was launched in 1998 with the mission of modernising medical education throughout the UK and the aim of improving healthcare.
- The services are offered free of charge to doctors and medical students in the UK.
- An integrated e-learning approach is provided, with online learning modules, discussion fora and personal development plans.
- Each learning module is case-based with a pre- and post-test MCQ.
- 40 000 doctors in the UK completed a quarter of a million online modules between 2001 and 2005.

Introduction

Doctors.net.uk was launched in 1998 with the mission of modernising medical education throughout the UK with the aim of improving healthcare. It delivers a comprehensive range of services that are free of charge to doctors and medical students. There are over 125 000 GMC-registered members, including 37 000 general practitioners (GPs).

e-learning: the drivers

Published in 2001, *Working Together – Learning Together* identified e-learning as a key part of the national agenda to modernise healthcare by shaping a workforce fit for the future.[1] Doctors.net.uk launched its electronic continuing medical education (eCME) programme that same year.

Amongst the factors driving e-learning are the emphasis on self-directed learning, the requirement for all doctors to plan and track their learning around a personal development plan (PDP) and constraints on the time and funding available to support all these activities.[2] Certainly, e-learning offers many and varied potential benefits, amongst which the British Learning Association numbers consistent delivery of programmes, flexibility to update and respond to change, low delivery costs for large numbers of learners, opportunities for learner involvement, opportunities to monitor and evaluate outcomes and, not least, access for all those who need it.[3]

Online learning by Doctors.net.uk

The Education section of the website developed as a natural progression of the medical information resources (databases, full-text journals and specialist pages) and communication tools (email and discussion fora) that Doctors.net.uk has provided since 1998 to help members find best evidence, communicate with their peers, reflect on their practice, share their knowledge and engage in professional debate.

Written by doctors, for doctors, the first online learning modules were launched in June 2001. Currently, more than 165 online learning modules are available, with new titles being added each month. The subject coverage spans the full range of skills needed in practice, from adult learning theory to painless visual loss, migraine to tax issues for GPs, life with Type 1 diabetes to sexually transmitted infections in men.

Partnerships

The unusual reach that the large membership of Doctors.net.uk affords is a powerful factor in attracting sponsors. Doctors.net.uk works with the Department of Health, the National Patient Safety Agency, the Health Protection Agency, the Royal Medical Colleges, other professional bodies and healthcare companies keen to support education and to engage doctors with key messages about clinical guidelines, best practice and patient safety.

e-learning offers a new medium through which healthcare organisations may effectively deliver these key messages and gain invaluable feedback from front-line staff.

Doctors.net.uk educational modules are independently authored and peer-reviewed to safeguard the provision of a highly respected educational resource.

An integrated learning resource

Doctors.net.uk provides an interactive and integrated medical education resource that is easily accessible and simple to use.

The *Education Guide* provides a simple overview of appraisal and revalidation, introduces e-learning and links to an online PDP (Personal Development Plan). This leads doctors through the process of assessing their professional development needs, enables them to record their learning activities and produce reports for appraisal. The web page automatically displays each module passed and stores the corresponding continuing professional development (CPD) certificates.

Each learning module links to relevant resources such as online journals, major textbooks (e.g. *The Oxford Textbook of Medicine*), Medline and e-formulary (giving up-to-date details on all UK drugs, dosages and monographs).

DocStore, a facility to store documents online, gives members the ability to keep records of clinical papers, photographs and other documents that support their learning and practice.

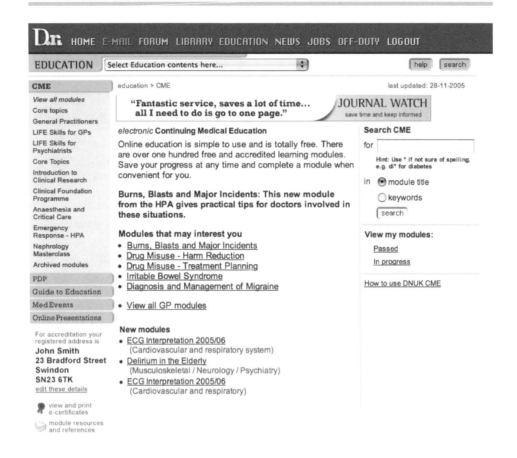

Figure 11.1 Entry portal to website

A community of practice

As a unique community of practice, exclusive to doctors, Doctors.net.uk facilitates informal and frank interaction between peers. More than 150 lively discussion fora are available in which members post comments and questions about best clinical practice. They learn from colleagues as they seek advice and information to guide the care of individual patients. Most modules link through to a discussion forum so that participants may reflect on their learning with their peers. Some groups use a 'closed' forum e.g. to support GPs undertaking a Postgraduate Certificate in Adult Education, and in these circumstances a coordinator is appointed to act as moderator.

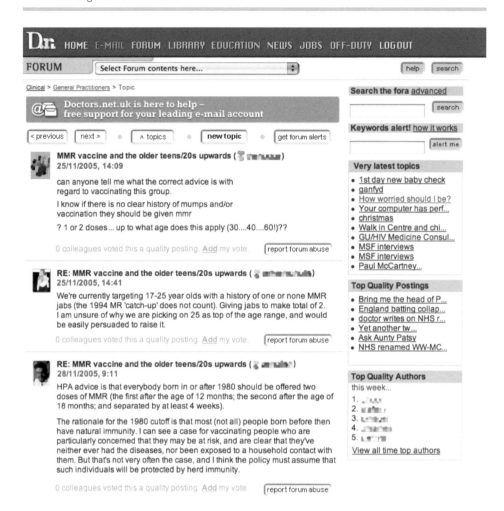

Figure 11.2 Discussion forum

Shaping the curriculum

The medical team tries to anticipate and respond to the learning needs of busy clinicians. New topics are frequently identified through member surveys as well as published reports, feedback from members and at the request of medical organisations, such as the Health Protection Agency. A survey of members in 2003 showed that only 6% of a sample of 200 GPs felt that they knew what to do in the event of a major incident.[4] In response, Doctors,net.uk was commissioned by the Health Protection Agency to develop and deliver an online training programme for doctors. Similarly, a report identifying that many junior doctors were unfamiliar with basic emergency medical care[5] led to collaboration with the National Electronic Library for Health to produce a training programme on the assessment and management of critical illness in Accident and Emergency departments.[6]

Aside from over 100 topics written specifically for GPs, modules are also provided for doctors in training, hospital consultants and all other grades.

Problem-centred

As outlined in the Doctors.net.uk module 'Learning effectively', Baxter explains the value of the case study approach; the experience of working through a patient's problems means that learners are 'more likely to recall the information when faced again with a patient'.[7]

The learning modules are based around patient scenarios to align the educational content with the challenges of real life. The scenarios serve as vehicles to impart short 'knowledge nuggets',[8] interactive, 'bite-sized' chunks of information on best practice in diagnosis and management, reflecting evidence-based clinical guidelines. The goal is to cover not only what action is appropriate but also to draw attention to action that is inappropriate. This is based on current evidence and guidelines.

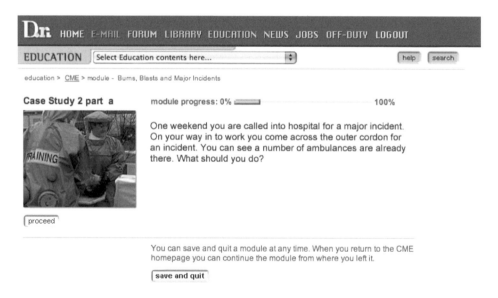

Figure 11.3 Learning module

Format and delivery

With minor variations, the learning modules always follow a standard format so that learners may benefit from a consistent interface and focus on the message. The common core components are:

- Introduction – including statement of learning objectives
- Pre-module test: Multiple Choice Questions (MCQ)
- Case Study 1
- Case Study 2

- Post-module MCQ (a repeat of the pre-test)
- Evaluation form
- Resource page.

Each case study is explored via a mix of text and graphics. Learners proceed through the case study, step by step, selecting a response to reflect their clinical decision at each stage. As each question is answered, text is displayed reflecting current guidelines and the best evidence available. A confirmation of their choice, or further explanation of factors to be considered, is then displayed. Finally, each module concludes with a resource page linking to further reading and activities.

There has been a deliberate decision to avoid 'flashy' technology which may create unnecessary technical barriers for users, and so impede the learning experience. The learner is encouraged to focus on the message not the medium. Learners simply 'pause' their progress through a module if short of time or unexpectedly interrupted, and can resume their learning at any time.

Managing quality

The quality of the online educational experience relies not simply on ensuring high standards of content and delivery of each component of an integrated mix of media, but also on ensuring seamless navigation between them. Thus, the education team manages quality in terms of content development, design, production and technical delivery, and the relationships between these. New modules are submitted for accreditation to the relevant professional body, piloted and revised on a regular basis.

Authoring

Writers are commissioned to reflect the latest clinical guidelines from authoritative sources and to use the best evidence available along with providing basic definitions, facts and figures. The focus is on the behaviour, attitudes, skills and knowledge most relevant to current practice. The vast majority of modules are written by busy clinicians who have hands-on experience of the subject in question. Where appropriate, for instance for a module on financial management, external experts are brought in.

Authors enjoy some flexibility and self-expression in the structure of the module, in relation to the length of the MCQ, the number of case studies used and the use of illustrations, figures and tables.

Peer review, monitoring and feedback

Peer review is key to the quality assurance process and Doctors.net.uk is fortunate to be able to draw on the expertise, interests and experience of members to create, review and revise learning materials.

Each new module is subject to peer review, as well as being checked by members of the medical team at Doctors.net.uk, to ensure that the material is relevant, robust and user-friendly. New modules are checked by the editorial team for technical bugs, before and after the module 'goes live'. Further, qualitative feedback from doctors who have completed the module is monitored at routine intervals.

Accreditation

Modules are accredited by the UK Conference of Educational Advisers, the Educational Providers Accreditation Scheme for Scotland (EPASS), the Royal College of Physicians (London) and the Royal College of Anaesthetists.

Usage of Doctors.net.uk learning modules

The online modules are a very popular resource.[8] In just over four years, between June 2001 and August 2005, almost 40 000 doctors in the UK successfully completed a quarter of a million modules totalling almost half a million hours of accredited learning between them. Just under 15 000 GPs are responsible for more than half of this number and they have undertaken more than a quarter of a million hours of accredited learning over this period. There are a number of real enthusiasts whose activity is astonishing. More than 1200 members have achieved passes in 30 or more modules and six members have completed more than 200 modules each.

Incident management for GPs, a module developed in partnership with the Health Protection Agency, was the single most popular module amongst GPs during this period.[9] With a pass rate of 82%, it was successfully completed, in 12 months, by 2705 doctors. Modules on osteoporosis and obesity were the two runners-up (passed by 2227 and 2057 doctors, respectively).

Evaluation of Doctors.net.uk learning modules

Recognising that it is almost impossible to demonstrate positive patient outcomes, which is the ultimate test for any educational intervention, Doctors.net.uk seeks to measure the acquisition of knowledge, increased awareness and confidence and user satisfaction as surrogate outcomes. The collection of these data, via MCQs, an online questionnaire and free-text feedback, has been automated to meet the needs of both members and sponsors for feedback on educational outcomes.

A report on the usage of a single learning module for GPs (on irritable bowel syndrome) between August 2001 and June 2004 has already been published.[10] The data clearly demonstrate that this approach satisfies the CRISIS criteria for continuing education. Effective provision must be Convenient, Relevant, Individual, Self-assessed, Inexpensive and take a Systematic approach.[11] The second 'I' in the mnemonic has been subject to some changes as the criteria have been reworked over the years, and Harden now focuses on the importance of Independent learning.[12]

The pass mark

The pass mark for UKCEA accredited modules is 70%; and 80% for those accredited by the Royal College of Physicians (London).

Table 11.1 reports activity for the 10 modules most popular with GPs in the 12 months between April 2004 and March 2005. Across these favourite modules, the pass rate varied from 82% to 95%.

Table 11.1 Most popular modules for GPs April 2004–March 2005

Subject	Starts	Passes	Pass %	Fails	Pending
Incident management for GPs	3308	2705	81.77	149	454
Diagnosis and management of osteoporosis	2344	2227	95.01	10	107
Management of obesity	2234	2057	92.08	26	151
Managing menorrhagia – initial steps	2160	2048	94.81	4	108
Irritable bowel syndrome	2168	1938	89.39	24	206
Diagnosis and management of migraine	1848	1760	95.24	6	82
Hypertension	1884	1696	90.02	1	187
Appraisal	1861	1616	86.84	10	235
Child health surveillance	1601	1517	94.75	7	77
Managing erectile dysfunction in general practice	1635	1506	92.11	16	113

The shift in MCQ test scores

The shift in pre-module and post-module test scores is taken as the key indicator of whether learners have gained and retained knowledge in the short term. The pre-test MCQ score is displayed immediately, giving doctors a clear indication of the currency of their knowledge before they begin to work through the module. At the end of the module, the post-test provides an opportunity to consolidate new knowledge and gives an indicator of short-term recall of new knowledge.

Table 11.2 Improvement in test scores: most popular modules Aug 2004–July 2005

Title	Passes	Pass %	Pre-score	Post-score	Improvement pre–post-test
Drug misuse – harm reduction	2865	84.12	70.56	84.48	13.92
Drug misuse – treatment planning	2011	86.94	67.88	82.01	14.13
Restless legs syndrome	1111	64.29	59.91	76.38	16.47
Incident management	1455	84.64	71.93	87.64	15.71
Tax issues for general practitioners	712	58.84	67.38	88.61	21.23
Overall	8154	75.77	67.53	83.82	16.29

Across the five most popular modules in a 12-month period, Table 11.2 reports an overall mean improvement of 16% in the post-module MCQ test, following completion of the module, varying from 14% to 21%. The pre-module test serves several purposes. It can enhance motivation, helping doctors to identify their learning needs while stimulating the individual to trawl information from long-term memory and bring it into short-term memory. Research suggests that learners who activate their prior knowledge can absorb twice as much new information on a topic as those who do not.[7] The MCQ format may also stimulate people to form their own questions and by activating prior knowledge in this way, they read more effectively and learn more efficiently.[7]

User satisfaction

Participants are asked to complete an online evaluation at the end of each module, rating how well it met the specified learning objectives and how user-friendly the materials were. They are asked to assess the effectiveness of the resource, for instance in terms of awareness of the condition and of treatments, increased confidence in diagnosis and ability to manage patients and enhanced knowledge, as well as to rate the user-friendliness of the materials. This evaluation form generates quantitative data that illuminate the perceptions of learners. Participants are also given an opportunity to feed back their own comments on the module.

Using the Irritable Bowel Syndrome (IBS) module (between August 2001 and July 2003) as an example, 97% of the 1936 doctors who submitted a post-module evaluation questionnaire rated the module as effective or very effective.

Overall, 99% of respondents who had taken the IBS module considered it user-friendly, highlighting that these users are comfortable with using the technology and are not experiencing technical barriers.[10]

Free-text feedback indicated that doctors taking the IBS module welcomed the ease of access and flexibility of e-learning, were pleased to be able to set their own pace, liked the design of the module and welcomed the opportunity to identify personal learning needs. There is an implication that doctors bring similar expectations to e-learning modules as they might to a GP refresher course, looking to review their knowledge and checking for gaps as well as to reinforce confidence in their knowledge base and improve their practice. Where there is any disappointment with the content, this is generally a result of those with greater than average initial knowledge of the particular subject wanting a greater challenge.[10]

Technical difficulties with using e-CME are unusual, and easily rectified. The Helpdesk team can also advise anyone who experiences local difficulties with connectivity.

Conclusion

Drawing on data gathered from the 40 000 doctors in the UK who completed a quarter of a million online modules between August 2001 and August 2005, users are very satisfied with the Doctors.net.uk approach to e-learning as a means to increase their knowledge, awareness and confidence. The sheer scale of the uptake indicates the potential power of e-learning as a vehicle for change, able to bypass organisational and geographical barriers to delivering medical education programmes across the UK.

The Doctors.net.uk model is already beginning to make real Harden's vision for distance learning and continuing medical education, using new learning technologies to provide physicians with learning opportunities and resources when and where they are required.[12] The challenge ahead is to make the move from delivering e-CME 'just in time' to offering personalised learning opportunities 'just for you'.

References

1 Department of Health (2001) *Working Together – Learning Together: a framework for lifelong learning for the NHS*. Department of Health, London.
2 Sandars J (2004) The e-learning site. *Education for Primary Care*. **15**: 117–18.
3 10 steps to getting started in e-learning (2003) British Learning Association. www. british-learning.com/home.htm.
4 National survey of general practitioners in the UK (2003) doctors.net.uk. November 2003.
5 Smith GB and Poplett N (2002) Knowledge of aspects of acute care amongst trainee doctors. *Postgraduate Medical Journal*. **78**: 335–8.
6 Ringrose T and Toth B (2003) Proof of the proposition. Rapid response. *BMJ*. 1 February 2003. http://bmj.bmjjournals.com/cgi/eletters/326/7382/176#29304.
7 Baxter C-M (2005) Learning efficiently – applying cognitive psychology to medical education. doctors.net.uk.
8 Lacey Bryant S and Ringrose T (2004) Doctors.net.uk education: GP usage of e-learning modules. *Work Based Learning in Primary Care*. **2**: 362–5.
9 Ruggles R and Ringrose T (2005) Go in, stay in, log in – developing an online module for incident management training for general practitioners. *Chemical Hazards and Poisons Report*. **4**: 46–7.
10 Lacey Bryant S and Ringrose T (2005) Evaluating the Doctors.net.uk model of electronic continuing medical education. *Work Based Learning in Primary Care*. **3**: 129–42.
11 Dunn WR and Hamilton DD (1986) Determining the continuing education priorities for pharmacists. *Pharmaceutical Journal*. **237**: 225–8.
12 Harden RM (2005) A new vision for distance learning and continuing medical education. *Journal of Continuing Education for Health Professionals*. **25**(1): 43–51.

Chapter 12

Becoming an e-tutor

Maura Murphy

Key points

- Preparation is essential to become an effective e-tutor.
- An e-tutor will be able to facilitate and support the future continuing education of local GPs to enable appraisal and revalidation.
- An e-tutor requires a range of skills, many of which are required to be an effective GP postgraduate tutor.
- An important aspect of the role of an e-tutor is giving feedback in order to motivate the learner.

Introduction

In this chapter I describe my experiences of undertaking the 'Certificate in e-Learning Tutoring Skills'. This certificate for training e-tutors is awarded by the Institute of IT Training which is a division of the National Computing Centre. The Approved Training Provider is The Training Foundation as part of their Certified e-Learning Professional Programme.

What is an e-tutor?

An e-tutor is responsible for supporting e-learners. This can be done in several ways depending on the individual situation.

Box 12.1 The four roles of the e-tutor

- administrator
- subject expert
- coach
- assessor

The e-tutor as administrator

Certain actions are necessary for the tutor to organise learners, arrange events and to maintain records. The following activities are characteristic of the tutor as administrator:

- registering new learners
- arranging learners into groups
- organising times for group events
- recording learner progress.

The e-tutor as subject expert

Not all of the content of a course can always be contained within the online materials. The tutor will often have a role to play in supplementing these materials. The following activities are characteristic of the tutor as subject expert: developing lists of frequently asked questions (FAQs); providing answers to questions on the material; delivering online lessons; and referring learners to resources.

The e-tutor as coach

Particularly with longer courses, a higher proportion of learners will require ongoing support and encouragement to help them through. The tutor has an important role to play as coach, responding to emerging needs of learners and acting as a listening post. The following activities are characteristic of the tutor as coach: chasing up learners who are falling behind schedule; encouraging learners and recognising their successes; counselling learners who are experiencing difficulties; and initiating activities that will help learners to progress towards their own goals and course objectives.

The e-tutor as assessor

Often it is the case that the achievements of the objectives of the course cannot be wholly measured using quizzes, simulations and other online self-study activities. The following activities are characteristic of the tutor as assessor: ensuring learners undergoing assessments are who they say they are; reviewing and judging assignments submitted by learners; 'observing' the actions of learners; and providing learners with specific, timely feedback.

   The required competencies to be an effective e-tutor are very similar for those required to be a postgraduate GP tutor. However, extra IT skills are necessary, as is the requirement to have access to the correct equipment, which works at the right time! The most important attribute of any tutor is good communication skills.

Box 12.2 The 12 principal competencies for e-tutors

1 Establish relationships with new learners.
2 Communicate appropriately with learners.
3 Provide administrative support.
4 Provide learners with technical and subject matter expertise.
5 Initiate activities that will facilitate learning.
6 Provide learners with support and encouragement.
7 Assess learners' performance.

8 Use web pages for communication with and between learners.
9 Use email for communication with learners.
10 Use bulletin boards and discussion forums for communication with and between learners.
11 Use text, audio and video conferencing for communication with and between learners.
12 Evaluate and continuously improve online tutoring support.

What makes an effective e-tutor?

Good organisational skills

Sufficient organisational skills are necessary to be able to keep track of what learners are doing and when to successfully co-ordinate events and to set up folders to store email correspondence. A chaotic or impulsive tutor will make too many mistakes and infuriate their learners, who, at a distance, will be less forgiving than in a face-to-face teaching situation.

Computer literacy

Learners depend on their tutor knowing their way around the web, email and conferencing software. Many students will be relative newcomers to these tools and will need guidance to sort out the inevitable teething problems involved in communicating online. A technophobic tutor will simply never get their course up and running.

Reliability

Learners rely on the tutor to be available when they say they will be and to respond within agreed timeframes. A person whose job means that they never know where they will be, and when, will find it hard to provide the sort of service learners will expect.

Articulate

e-tutors spend a great deal of their time at their computer writing. They must be sufficiently articulate to write clearly and unambiguously. The 'stream of consciousness' writer will seriously confuse their students.

Learner-centred

It pays to be learner-centred in the classroom. It is even more important online. It is not the place of the tutor to dominate, to tell, sell or dictate. The best tutors are facilitators, creating an environment in which learners can prosper on their own initiative as independent, hopefully lifelong, learners.

Concise

Unless you are a fast typist, the process of communicating the written word can be extremely time-consuming. The verbose tutor will consume so much time in routine communication that they will not be able to cope – they will also run away with the budget! e-tutors will thus benefit from being able to touch-type.

Friendly

It can be a lonely existence for the e-learner and it is important that the tutor compensates for this with a bit of humanity. A warm, accessible tutor with a good sense of humour will soon become a student's best friend. A cold, intimidating one will soon end up as lonely as their students.

Knowledgeable

Learners will expect the tutor to know more than them and to be able to resolve any misunderstandings with the material. It is not essential to be an absolute expert on the course content.

Imaginative

In the role of coach, a tutor will need to respond to emergent and sometimes unpredictable learner needs. Coming up with suggestions for activities that will overcome obstacles and move students on towards the objectives are another necessary skill for a tutor. With a little imagination, the course will not be the same every time – it will respond creatively to the inevitable differences in the learners.

Firm

Learning is not all fun. Sometimes the tutor will have to deal firmly with students who break the rules, who upset other learners or who fail to deliver on their promises. And if passing the course is to have any real meaning, there will be times when the tutor will have to mark low or even remove a learner from the course. If the tutor is weak, the learners will not respect this.

The e-tutor training programme

Once logged on to the programme website there was a home page with access to all the course material, with a notice board in the middle of the page to keep everyone updated with events such as forthcoming chats. The main part for course materials, including a course manual, was in the Learn Online section. Most communication between participants and the tutor occurred in Messenger, where emails landed daily from the tutor and group. There was also a help facility and a calendar facility.

The forums were a section in which group discussions took place. Participants worked in small groups (usually six) and were expected to join in a chat every week. One of the group acted as a host each week and picked a topic. The group met up online at an agreed time and date. Trying to greet and welcome everyone, carrying on the chat with the others and summarising the contributions was quite a skill to acquire. It was really just small group work online but I could not afford to lose my concentration. At the end we wrote our farewells and then the host saved the chat. This was then emailed to the tutor and also sent to everyone in the group. The tutor then marked this in our personal area on the website and we could read the feedback and learn from this. It was exciting and became addictive!

There were three assignments, one for each module, and these included tests online and various activities e.g. hosting a web chat. It was very clearly set out and any problems could soon be sorted with our tutor via Messenger or email; the telephone was used in emergencies!

The modules

Box 12.3 The modules

The e-learning primer: 10 hours over 2 weeks
e-tutoring methods: 12 hours over 2 weeks
e-tutoring skills: 26 hours over 6 weeks

---

e-learning primer

This was the first module of the course which explained the benefits of e-learning. Adding e-learning to the mix of learning methods was discussed. Web pages, internet speeds, web technologies and browsers were all contained in the downloaded manual so that we could learn from it in order to answer the questions put in our assignments.

e-tutoring methods

This was the next module on the course and it commenced by discussing 'Who needs a website?' If the course consists of more than just interactive materials for personal study, then using a website is one way to communicate with your students. Other methods are audio tapes, videos, CD-ROMs, books and TV broadcasts. A website is also an extremely low-cost method for communicating, if necessary, over long distances. Conclusions as to what should be on a website were:

- frequently asked questions, including a list of answers
- contact details
- listings – web links, books, journal articles, videos or any other study material
- course materials – providing access to these for downloading or viewing online
- facilities – e.g. conferencing, text-based chat and asynchronous discussion.

The importance of email was discussed and I learnt that the Queen started emailing in 1976! Few academics were this far-sighted!

It was suggested that these were the advantages of email:

- Your audience gets your message personally.
- You want a quick but not an instant response.
- You want time to compose your message.
- You require a record of your message.

Don't use email when:

- You need an immediate response.
- You are delivering sensitive information.
- Text is not a powerful enough medium so you may need graphics, video or audio.
- You are agitated! This is e-rage and it is not good for your career so it is better to kick the cat!

From the above it can be seen that asynchronous discussions (discussions online which are not held at the same time) were not always helpful, and the necessity for some synchronous discussions, such as live chats, came through on the course. The tutor should establish the rules of communication and explain the mechanics of using the software. The tutor suggests to the students the sorts of topics that would be suitable for discussion, how new topics are initiated, any issues of netiquette and any rules for acceptable behaviour. If a student breaks the rules then the tutor must bring this to the notice of the student by telephone and redirect him or her.

Synchronous discussion may be used when:

- An instant response is necessary.
- An issue must be resolved immediately.
- Seeing and hearing each other is important.
- A message needs to get through and an answer obtained immediately.

In our course the tutor controlled any discussions that were straying off course by using Messenger. Outcomes were summarised by the tutor at each stage of the discussion. Archiving only genuinely useful messages and deleting irrelevant messages was also the duty of the tutor.

The mechanics of synchronous discussion were then explained. Text chat was the most basic of the synchronous methods and the easiest to implement. Electronic whiteboards, audio conferencing, video conferencing, application sharing and polling were also explained in detail.

The tutor could help to manage synchronous discussions as follows:

- by establishing the rules of communication
- by communicating the goal and the timeframe
- by encouraging everyone to contribute
- by controlling discussions so that they do not stray off course
- by summarising at each stage of the discussion
- by acting against any misuse of the facility.

e-tutoring skills

This was the most interesting and most difficult module. In the classroom it was possible to tell a lot about a new student from their appearance, manner of speaking and behaviour, whereas online this was not possible. It is essential to identify:

- basic details-name, age, gender/sex etc.
- contact information – by email, phone and perhaps surface mail
- current job
- education and career history
- prior knowledge and expertise
- the level of computer literacy
- the goals of the student
- the students' preferred learning styles
- obstacles – personal, occupational or sickness.

The students will also appreciate information about the tutor, including the obvious basic details, such as contact information, education and career history.

The Learning Contract was then explained: an agreement between the tutor and the learner aiming to secure positive learning. Clear examples of good practice in drawing up contracts were shown. Many of the other subjects in this module have already been covered in the section on how to be an effective tutor. A very clear outline of how to deliver real-time lessons was very helpful – preparation was everything! The nature of motivation was included in 'Helping learners to set goals'; motivation was a function of two factors: the desirability of rewards and the feasibility of achieving those rewards. The tutor as coach could do much to influence students' motivation and prevent them from dropping out of the course.

Providing students with feedback was the last part of this module. Rules for effective feedback were laid out as this was crucial to continuing motivation.

The students on our course then had to write a report in which examples of problems and resolutions were given and discussed. The students also had to give peer feedback to a course colleague (a 'buddy') about their chat and this was found to be very helpful and positive.

Box 12.4 Helpful hints

- Motivate yourself to learn.
- Be willing to change your attitudes.
- Keep your mind open to new ideas which may improve the lives of patients and doctors.
- Consider becoming an 'e-missionary'. (A missionary is one who is sent by a higher authority to open the minds of the unknowing!)
- Be accurate, clear and brief when giving feedback.

Further information

The Training Foundation, Foundation House, Milburn Hill Road, University of Warwick Science Park, Coventry CV4 7EZ.
email: info@trainingfoundation.com
Web: www.trainingfoundation.com

Chapter 13

Running a short course on e-learning – a GP tutor's perspective

Peter Johnson

Key points

- Familiarise yourself with local e-resources and their availability if you are considering running a course.
- The three main areas to focus on when designing a course on e-learning are: instructional design principles, the educational media and evaluation.
- The design phase of any e-learning course is of equal importance as the e-learning materials (graphics, content and text).
- Constantly evaluate the course at each stage of its development.

Introduction

Running a course on e-learning, at first, may seem a daunting prospect; it was for me initially when I was asked to develop a short course for GP non-principals. How to deal with the technology? What if something goes wrong? I believe that so long as we use the same general educational principles that are applied to other courses, with a few considerations for e-learning, then there should be few problems.

The design phase of any course is important in its development.[1] Time and effort invested at this stage can help avert any future problems; this is especially true for e-learning. e-learning media are so noticeable in terms of graphics, content and text. They are highly visible to public scrutiny.

In this chapter, I hope to give some guidance as to what I see as important when designing and running a course either on, or involving, some e-learning. I intend to focus on the three areas that I feel will help educators the most when considering using e-learning, namely, instructional design, educational media and evaluation.

Some practical considerations

Upon deciding to run a course on e-learning it is worth firstly considering some practical issues. These would include how and where the course is to be held? Are there any local computer facilities you can use? If so, how many computers are available and do they have online high speed connections? Will you be posting elements of your course on the internet and if so do you have the expertise with web design? Will these web-based activities be synchronous or asynchronous activities? Will you be using a blended learning approach?

I would strongly recommend discovering and familiarising yourself with the availability of resources to you in your locality, and considering which elements of these you would use in your course design.

Course design: general considerations

Some have stated that traditional instructional design principles are misapplied or used in justification of designs that do not work, and that with regards to e-learning these should be abandoned.[2] I do not agree with this assertion, since e-learning uses different forms of media, and these design principles apply to any other form of *educational media* – be that a handout, computer software or a PowerPoint presentation. It is important to be aware when examining e-learning material not to be fooled by a glossy or glitzy appearance, but to take care to determine the educational value of the material to be used. Close attention should therefore be given during the design phase of a course to potential media to be used; design *then* technology, not the reverse. This is particularly true if a blended-learning (i.e. mixed methods) approach is to be used.

Instructional design is a process of organising learning resources to assist learners in their achievement of educational goals. It is a process to ensure that learning does not occur in a haphazard manner, creating a 'framework'. The course designer should create an instructional experience that ensures the learners achieve their objectives. Instructional design in e-learning should attempt to link educational theory with the technology, making the learning and not the technology the centre of its development. The use of instructional design principles with e-learning can help prevent any misapplication of technology to educational theory or methods. Aspects of technology, no matter how good or advanced, cannot make up for poor design. Educators and course designers play a pivotal role in the linking of technology with the relevant educational theory.

There are many models of instructional design; I intend to present a well known and frequently used method for instructional design – the ADDIE model. This model is a general and systematic approach to the instructional design process. It provides a structure for educators to ensure their instruction is effective and creative both in the design and development of a course. ADDIE stands for: Analyse, Design, Develop, Implement and Evaluate. This label does not appear to have been claimed by a single author, but has evolved as a generic model and developed from others.

Each element of the model is a vital part of the instructional design process, and careful attention should be maintained throughout. The following is a summary of important elements of each phase; it is not exhaustive but should give you an outline of the process. I have adapted these with e-learning elements of a course in mind.

The analysis phase

- Who is the audience?
- What are their educational needs and wants?
- What are the delivery options? – www/CD/WAP/computer laboratory/blended learning approach.
- What constraints are there? – Time, money/resources/facilitators/tutors/e-tutors.
- Problem identification – reflect and identify areas where problems may arise.
- When is the course to be run?
- When will it be completed?

The design phase

- Consider and define the educational objectives of the course.
- Determine the sequencing of all elements of the course, and how they might integrate with other learning.
- Establish an overall style to the course in terms of how it will look and feel – be consistent with the design elements.
- Consider and reflect on **all** forms of educational media.
- Evaluate the media and choose those that best fit with the course objectives.
- If e-learning elements have been chosen – then consider how these will be used, how learners will access the e-learning material and how problems might be solved (IT support).
- Identify resources.
- Integration – how will the course integrate with other work and learning?
- Make the learning process as interactive as possible.

The development phase

- Create or obtain the required educational media.
- Determine how learners will interact with each other and the media.
- Consider any hardware/software issues that may arise during the course.
- Consider a venue for the course.
- Plan out the sequencing of learning throughout the course.
- Have a back-up plan ready in the event of technical problems.
- Consider and develop an evaluation strategy.

The implementation phase

- Distribute pre-course materials.
- Double-check that all elements of the course have been looked after.
- Make sure one person leads on a specific area to avoid omissions and or duplication.

The evaluation phase

- Implement your evaluation strategy.
- How are you going to focus your evaluation?
- In light of information gathered, reflect and loop back to the analysis phase.

Although the 'ADDIE' model for instructional design is generic, it is adaptable to the e-learning situation and process. It focuses the course designer on key areas for consideration. I found it an invaluable resource to helping me design a course about e-learning for non-principals. During the process this model can highlight areas where problems may arise. Thus, some focused thought in the design/ development process can improve the courses feel and structure and hence enhance the students' learning experience.

Educational media

The term 'media' as in 'educational media' can be interpreted as the means by which something is communicated. The communication of facts, information, attitudes, ethics etc. can all be done with a number of 'media'. Aspects we should consider when developing course media are – who and what is it for? How will it be used? What are the practicalities? Designing and using various educational media therefore has important implications; whatever media is chosen must be initially explored with reference to educational theory and the course objectives.

Comments on the function of instructional text with medical education have included that its success demands 'attention to the content as well as the way it is presented'.[3]

Much has been written about instructional text. In terms of language and readability, structure and organisation and the use of illustrations.[3–6] Far less has been written in relation to e-learning media, although some issues may be readily transferable. Ruth Clark, in the *e-learning Developers Journal* (online journal) wrote about 'Six Principles of Effective e-learning: What Works and Why?'[7] It gives us some guidance on what to consider when designing or using e-learning material.

1 **The Multimedia Principle: adding graphics to words can improve learning:** This is certainly true and backed up by other research; however, it may also distract the reader.[6] Simple illustrations are often the best and probably committed to memory first and retained longer than printed text.[4]
2 **The Contiguity Principle: placing text near graphics improves learning:** Consider using a scrolling screen where an illustration and text cannot be seen together as they are set above and below each other, it is far better to position then side by side. Once again, this is supported by some instructional text work.[4]
3 **The Modality Principle:** Explaining graphics with audio can improve learning. The assertion here is that visual processing of information is supported by phonetic processing.
4 **The Redundancy Principle:** Explaining graphics with audio and redundant text can interfere with learning. Learning can actually be suppressed when a graphic is explained by a combination of text and narration reading the same text. With this combination there is simply too much information to process.
5 **The Coherence Principle:** Using gratuitous visuals, text and sounds can interfere with learning. Clark asserts that this tells us 'Less is More', especially when learning is the primary goal. This is similar to the acronym KISS: keep it simple.
6 **The Personalisation Principle:** Use conversational tone and pedagogical agents to increase learning. I think care needs to be taken here as some

language in the first and second person may come across as condescending or too simple.[8] This may also be true with pedagogical agents (onscreen coaches that help learners negotiate and mediate e-learning programmes e.g. 'Merlin' – Microsoft Office's Assistant), especially when our e-learning 'clients' are all adults; Clark's article includes reference to school-aged children.

In summary, aspects of media play an important role in motivating and aiding retention of information of learners. Learning should always remain the central focus for any designer or user of e-learning material, a glitzy approach distracts from the central learning message.

Evaluation

Evaluation is an important aspect of education; it is unfortunately often an afterthought. e-learning in medical education is a fast-growing field; new developments such as m-learning (mobile learning) are emerging. There is, therefore, a need for the effectiveness of these new technologies and media to be evaluated; it will be up to us as educators to do so in an open-minded, non-biased way.

Evaluation should not just be about outcomes but be considered as an integral part of any course development.[8] Sadly it is often thought of at a late stage, often leading to a mismatch of evaluation method and course design. Careful consideration should therefore be given to evaluation in the design phase of any course planning. It is important to be aware of the need for evaluation planning from the outset.

There have been many evaluation models reported; perhaps the one that could help us most is Stufflebeam's 'CIPP' approach which looks at several areas in evaluation.[9] The Context (the *intended outcomes*), the Input (the *intended means* i.e. programme strategy), the Process (the *actual means* of implementation of the programme strategy) and the Product (the *actual outcomes* of the programme). It is thorough and provides a framework to specify areas for evaluation.[10] It is possible to do either a broad evaluation across all aspects of the CIPP approach or to focus in on one or two of the aspects. Equally the course itself could be evaluated as a whole or looked at with regards to specific areas.

A useful method of determining the depth of your evaluation is to utilise a hierarchy such as that developed by Kirkpatrick.[11] Others have commented that this approach could be used and adapted to community educational evaluations.[12]

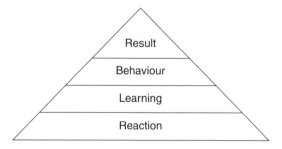

Figure 13.1 Kirkpatrick's hierarchy

The base of the hierarchy involves attaining the *reaction* of programme participants and an estimate of learner satisfaction e.g. were participants satisfied with the course? This level probably accounts for most evaluations done at the end of a course. The next level relates to *actual learning*, where the evaluator collects data on the new knowledge/skills learners can demonstrate e.g. can participants demonstrate their acquisition of skills? The third level is concerned with the *transference of behaviour learned* in the learning environment to real-life settings e.g. are the skills used at work? Finally, the highest level concerns the *broad impact on the wider community* i.e. how has the new learning impacted on the wider community? The depth of evaluation is an important factor to consider as initial reactions to a course can be misleading. The hierarchy can be illustrated as shown in Figure 13.1.

A simple way of developing an evaluation is to firstly decide what to evaluate. This is the initial step in the approach recommended by Rotem and Bandaranayake for tackling what might otherwise become a complex activity.[13] It is a simple and logical approach, and can be adapted to an area of new development. The main difficulty is how to decide what we evaluate.

Box 13.1 Evaluation approach (after Rotem and Bandaranayake)[13]

- Step 1: Decide what to evaluate
- Step 2: Design the evaluation strategy
- Step 3: Conduct the evaluation
- Step 4: Analyse the data
- Step 5: Make decisions

Individuals will have their own evaluation criteria or questions that depend on the purpose and focus of the evaluation. These may come from an 'external' source (e.g. health authority, clinical governance) or from an 'internal' source (e.g. target standards).[14] Hence 'specific' criteria will vary between evaluations. Currently, little research evidence exists about the effectiveness of e-learning activity.[15] Recent reviews of outcomes of e-learning activity have shown that there is limited evidence for performance change in clinical practice, nor has there been any influence on patient or health outcomes.[16,17] Therefore, if we are running a course or using e-learning material we need to evaluate them.

Conclusion

The areas I have presented in this chapter are the three key areas that I believe we should focus on when considering using e-learning material. Good instructional design coupled with appropriate use of media allows us to provide quality e-learning material, but we must evaluate otherwise we will never really recognise good e-learning material, nor develop improved e-learning standards.

References

1 Quinn FM (1995) *The Principles and Practice of Nurse Education* (3e). Chapman and Hall, London.
2 Allen MW (2003) *Michael Allen's Guide to e-Learning*. Wiley, Cichester.
3 McLeod PJ (1991) How to produce instructional text for a medical audience. *Medical Teacher*. **13**(2): 135–44.
4 Brown G and Tomlinson D (1980) Improve handouts. *Medical Teacher*. **2**(5): 215–20.
5 MacLean I (1991) Twelve tips on providing handouts. *Medical Teacher*. **13**(1): 7–12.
6 Hartley J (1985) *Designing Instructional Text* (2e). Kogan Page, London.
7 Clark R (2002) Six principles of effective e-learning: what works and why. *The e-Learning Developers Journal*. **2002** (Sept): 1–8. www.usoe.k12.ut.us/curr/ednet/training/resources/pdf/SixPrinciples9112002.pdf.
8 Kelly AV (1989) *The Curriculum – Theory and Practice* (3e). Paul Chapman Publishing Ltd, London.
9 Stufflebeam FT, Foley WJ, Cuba BC *et al.* (1971) *Medical Evaluation and Decision-Making*. FE Peacock, Itasca.
10 Calder J (1994) *Programme Evaluation and Quality: a comprehensive guide to setting up an evaluation system*. Kogan Page, London.
11 Kirkpatrick DI (1967) Evaluation of training. In: R Craig and I Bittel. *Training and Development Handbook*. McGraw-Hill, New York.
12 Brookfield SD (1986) *Understanding and Facilitating Adult Learning*. Open University Press, Milton Keynes.
13 Rotem A and Bandaranayake R (1983) How to plan and conduct programme evaluation. *Medical Teacher*. **5**(4): 127–31.
14 Grol R and Lawrence M (1995) *Quality Improvement by Peer Review*. Oxford University Press, Oxford.
15 Wong G, Greenhalgh T, Russell J *et al.* (2003) Putting your course on the web: lessons from a case study and systematic literature review. *Medical Education*. **37**: 1020–23.
16 Curran VR and Fleet L (2005) A review of evaluation outcomes of web-based continuing medical education. *Medical Education*. **39**: 561–7.
17 Klass DJ (2004) Will e-learning improve clinical judgement? *BMJ*. **328**: 1147–8.

Chapter 14

The Web Quest approach to e-learning

John Sandars

Key points

- Web Quests offer a structured enquiry-orientated approach to learning.
- Extensive use is made of information resources from the internet.
- An important aspect is the development of transferable skills in retrieval and appraisal of information obtained from the internet.
- The Web Quest approach is highly applicable for trainers and course organisers, but also for continuing professional development.

Introduction

The internet offers a vast and ever-increasing range of information resources. A recent estimate suggested that there are now over 33 million websites and in excess of one billion web pages.[1] Most of these resources are free and available 'any time and any place'. 'Surfing the net', in which websites are accessed to meet self-directed learning needs, is a popular activity. In 2000, surfing by Canadian men at home was 11.5 hours a month.[2] Almost all healthcare professionals in the United Kingdom have access to the internet, either at home or at work, and two recent surveys of primary healthcare professionals note that they are making increasing use of it as a method for self-directed education but measures of the full extent are not available.[3,4]

The Web Quest approach uses internet resources as an essential, and integral, component of the learning method. In this chapter I describe the approach and offer suggestions on how it can be used by GP educators.

What is a Web Quest?

The guru of Web Quests is Bernie Dodge of the Educational Technology Department at San Diego State University. He defines a Web Quest as 'an inquiry-orientated activity in which some or all of the information that learners interact with comes from resources on the internet'.[5] The basic structure of a Web Quest was developed in 1995 and since that time several thousand have been developed and used by millions of learners throughout the world. Numerous examples are provided on Bernie Dodge's extensive website. All are from the area of primary or secondary education, with no examples of its use in further and higher education.

Box 14.1 The main components of a Web Quest

- Title
- Introduction
- Task
- Resources
- Conclusion

The structure of a Web Quest, as originally described, consists of several components. The teacher initially identifies a clearly defined area of study and a related task. This task requires the learner to perform several activities in which information is accessed from several websites. An important aspect of all Web Quests is to engage the learner in a task that elicits higher order thinking, rather than simple information searching and recall. These tasks should involve problem solving, judgement, synthesis and analysis of information. Another important aspect is working within a group of learners, thereby developing collaborative learning.

The Web Quest is usually presented as a printed sheet and given to a group of learners, with each learner working on a separate activity within the task. However, group members can have the same activities and occasionally a Web Quest can be only undertaken by an individual.

Writing a Web Quest

This requires a structured process:

- **Title:** This should provide a concise description of the Web Quest.
- **Introduction:** A short paragraph provides background information and context for the activity. The learning objectives can also be stated in this section.
- **Task:** The activities required by the learner/learners should be clearly described. For example, this may include a series of questions, a summary to be created or a problem to be solved.
- **Resources:** Key internet resources should be given, including the title and the URL and hyperlink.
- **Conclusion:** This summarises what the learner/learners are expected to have accomplished or learnt by completing the activity. Often there will be a question to stimulate further thought.

Box 14.2 Example of a Web Quest suitable for an individual learner

Title: Web Quest on teamwork

Introduction

Teams are important for the effective delivery of healthcare. However, a successful team does not suddenly exist. This Web Quest will help you to identify the main factors that are required to enable a team to work effectively and how a team can be developed.

Task

Please access all three online resources.
Each resource will give you a different perspective on team work.
After reading through all of the resources, consider:

- What is a team?
- What are the features of an effective team?
- What are the implications for building an effective team?
- What is the role of the individual in the team?

Resources

1 Allen G *Supervision*.
   http://ollie.dcccd.edu/mgmt1374/book_contents/4directing/teambldg/
   teambldg.htm.
2 Brearley M (2000) Teams: lessons from the world of sport. *BMJ*. **321**:
   1141–3 (4 November) http://bmj.bmjjournals.com/cgi/content/full/321/
   7269/1141.
3 Enock K *Organisation and Management of Healthcare: group theories*.
   www.phel.gov.uk/hkdocs/OMH%20Katie%20Enock%20-
   Group%20theories%202002.pdf.

Conclusion

On completion of this Web Quest, you should have a clear action plan on
how to develop your team. What is your action plan going to be?

Educational rationale of the Web Quest approach

The structure of a Web Quest closely follows Robert Gagne's theory of instruction.[6] Gagne proposes that there is a rational relationship between the
methods of instruction, their effects on the learning processes and the learning
outcomes that are produced. An important aspect of both this model and a Web
Quest is the use of a structured step-wise model. The expectation of this
structured approach is that increased learning will occur, rather than by simply
'surfing' of the internet.

An important aspect of a Web Quest is the use of collaborative activities to
enhance the learning experience. Collaboration produces increased learning for
both individual members of the group and the group as a whole.[7] The main
advantage of collaborative learning is that there is active sharing of information
and, in addition, there are often challenges to underlying beliefs and assumptions.

Enquiry-based methods are associated with increased comprehension and
learner satisfaction.[8] A key component of all Web Quests is the clear set of
activities that the learner is required to perform.

Two important transferable skills can be developed whilst undertaking a Web
Quest: retrieval of information from a website and the appraisal of information
obtained from a website.

The Web Quest approach to enhance GP education

The original Web Quest approach can be modified to ensure that it is more applicable to GP education. A trainer can develop a Web Quest suitable for an individual registrar, such as illustrated in Box 14.2, but it can also be used as a group activity for a vocational training scheme.

The modified approach can be used for continuing professional development, with the involvement of the interdisciplinary primary healthcare team. There can be joint identification of a topic and then subsequent collaborative activities. A fictional illustration is presented that highlights the educational potential.

Box 14.3 A fictional illustration of how a Web Quest can be developed and used by a primary healthcare team

Yearly educational appraisal for all practice staff was an important method to identify the learning needs of individual staff members, but also for the practice. An overall practice learning need about improving the care of older people with dementia was identified and a small group of healthcare professionals in the practice decided to develop and use a Web Quest for the next practice learning day.

Developing the Web Quest

One of the doctors mentioned that she had found a website that offered help in the diagnosis and treatment of dementia. This was provided by the Scottish Intercollegiate Guidelines Network (SIGN) (www.show.scot.nhs.uk/sign/guidelines/published/index.html).

The practice nurse stated that the practice needed to offer care that was a partnership between healthcare professionals, older people with dementia and their carers. She remembered a resource on the Royal College of Nursing website (www.rcn.org.uk/downloads/scotland/caring_partnership.pdf).

The practice manager was concerned about how the practice could ensure consistent information care to older people with dementia and their carers. Carers often asked the receptionists for information. He had already looked at the Alzheimer's Society website (www.alzheimers.org.uk).

It rapidly became apparent that neither the doctors, nurses or receptionists were aware of a 'good' source of patient and carer information, and that the doctors and nurses were unsure of the current trends in diagnosis and treatment.

A Web Quest was written in preparation for the practice learning day and this had two main tasks:

1 All members of the primary healthcare team would look at, and evaluate, the patient and carer information on the Alzheimer's Society website.
2 All the doctors and nurses of the primary healthcare team would look at, and evaluate, the advice on diagnosis and treatment that was provided on the three websites that had been identified by the small group.

Using the Web Quest

On the practice learning day, there was a focused discussion on the 'best' patient and carer information sheet. The doctors and nurses noted that the SIGN guideline was under review (since it was produced in 1998) but the Alzheimer's Society website offered more updated advice on current best diagnosis and treatment. The doctors and nurses also had a brisk discussion on the role of partnership working.

Evaluating the learning experience

The primary healthcare team reviewed the practice learning day, especially the use of the Web Quest. Everyone stated that they had found it extremely useful. Information could be obtained from several sources, then compared and synthesised. An important aspect was the interdisciplinary discussion between the various members of the primary healthcare team. In addition, everyone felt that it had increased their skills and interest in using web-based information resources. They were all eager to start another Web Quest.

Developing skills in website access and appraisal

Anybody can launch a website, and there is no overall control over the quality of its content. The information provided by a website can be excellent but it can also be poor, and even downright wrong or dangerous. However, there is an excellent free source of information. Virtual Salt is an excellent website that offers help in the access and appraisal of internet sources of information.[9]

The main appraisal criteria are:

- **Credibility:** It is important to consider the author's credentials and any evidence of a quality control system, such as origination from a peer-reviewed publication.
- **Accuracy:** A judgement of the timeliness of the presented information is essential since often websites are not frequently updated.
- **Reasonableness:** A good website should offer a balanced view of the available information.
- **Support:** This is concerned with the source and corroboration of the information.

Conclusion

The Web Quest approach offers an exciting method to enhance GP learning by providing a structured learning experience that utilises the vast repository of information based on the internet. There is a lack of firm evidence to support their effectiveness in improving learning, including additional benefit over self-directed 'surfing'. However, Web Quests are based on sound educational principles and there is a 'common sense' appeal to this approach. It is surprising that there has been no description of this approach in the healthcare education literature.

Useful resources

General information on the Web Quest approach

Bernie Dodge has an excellent website with numerous examples of how to develop effective Web Quests (http://webquest.sdsu.edu/).

Resources for use in a Web Quest

Google Scholar enables specific searches for scholarly literature, including peer-reviewed papers, theses, books, abstracts and technical reports from all broad areas of research (www.scholar.google.com/).

An excellent resource of medically related websites can be found at www.rsmpress.co.uk/bkkiley2.htm.

Internet search and appraisal skills

The Resource Discovery Network Virtual Training Suite (www.vts.rdn.ac.uk/) is a set of free online tutorials designed to help students and lecturers improve their skills in the search and appraisal of internet sources of information. Users can work at their own pace and there are quizzes and interactive exercises to lighten the learning experience. An important feature of this resource is that there are separate tutorials for a range of healthcare, social care and management professionals.

References

1 Forrest E (2003) *Internet Marketing Intelligence*. McGraw-Hill Higher Education, New York.
2 www.mediaawareness.ca/english/resources/research_documents/statistics/internet/canadians_hooked_web.cfm [accessed 15 February 2005].
3 Wilson SM (1999) Impact of the internet on primary care staff in Glasgow. *Journal of Medical Internet Research*. 1: 1–12.
4 Moffat MO, Moffat KJ and Cano V (2001) General practitioners and the internet – a questionnaire survey of internet connectivity and use in Lothian. *Health Bulletin*. 59(2): 120–26.
5 www.webquest.sdsu.edu/ [accessed 15 February 2005].
6 Gagne RM (1985) *The Conditions of Learning and Theory of Instruction*. Holt, Rinehart and Winston, New York.
7 Jarvis P (1995) *Adult and Continuing Education*. Routledge, London.
8 Wiley J and Voss J (1999) Constructing arguments from multiple sources: tasks that promote understanding and not just memory for text. *Journal of Educational Psychology*. 91(2): 301–11.
9 www.virtualsalt.com/evalu8it.htm [accessed 15 February 2005].

Chapter 15

Experiences of an online learning network for GP continuing professional development

John Sandars and Michele Langlois

Key points

- Online learning networks for GPs offer an exciting opportunity to share knowledge and learn from one another.
- An online network for GP continuing professional development is described that offered a structured approach, with initial socialisation and action learning set-type activities.
- There was a low level of online network activity and the online discussions were superficial.
- Trust between the members of the online network was low and this inhibited online discussion.
- The results of the evaluation are similar to those for other online learning networks in a variety of settings.

Introduction

An important aspect of continuing professional development (CPD) for general practitioners (GPs) is the opportunity to share knowledge and learn together.[1] Recent developments in information and communication technology (ICT) have increased these opportunities, enabling groups of widely dispersed individuals to form online learning networks.[2] There is current interest in the National Health Service (NHS) for both the use of online learning and networks for CPD.[3,4] At the same time there has been investment in the supporting ICT infrastructure.[5] However, there has been little development of online learning networks for CPD within the NHS.

In this chapter, we describe our experience of the implementation and evaluation of a pilot online learning network for a group of GPs who worked in an inner-city area of north-west England (NW). This case study is the first United Kingdom (UK) study to describe an online learning network for GPs that was specifically designed to be used as a model for CPD.

The educational and technical aspects of the online learning network

The online network was hosted as an asynchronous discussion board within a dedicated website and used WebCT as the learning platform (www.webct.com). An asynchronous approach allows messages to be posted and read over a period of time, compared with a real-time synchronous approach.[6] The discussion board consisted of 10 structured activities. The importance of initial socialisation to encourage the formation of trust, an important prerequisite to enable knowledge sharing, was recognised and the first four structured activities were designed to facilitate introductions and share concerns about using the discussion board.[7] The rest of the structured activities used an action learning set-type of approach, which allowed members of the network to share knowledge about a mutually agreed topic and then to consider what important lessons could be used in the future.[8] Action learning sets have the potential to bring people together to find solutions to problems and, at the same time, lead to individual development.[9] Each activity was introduced by a facilitator and remained open for two weeks, enabling the members to use the discussion board in a logical sequence. Regular email prompts were sent to remind members when a new activity was open. Online facilitation was provided (JS) and a dedicated technology support line was offered (ML).

Evaluation of the online learning network

The evaluation had three main objectives:

1 Identification of the perceptions of participants to the use of an online learning network, both before and after entry to the network.
2 Identification of the processes that occur when an online learning network is used.
3 Identification of the impact on practice following participation in an online learning network.

Originally 23 GPs agreed to join and were registered on the online learning network but only 15 members actually entered the online network. Five were regular and consistent contributors.

Main findings

Technical and information retrieval skills

The majority of registered participants seemed relatively at ease with ICT, with 14 (93%) enjoying the experience of going online and 12 (80%) going online at least three days a week. Only one member stated that they had any prior experience of being involved in an online network. There was no significant difference before and after entering the online network.

Communication, assistance and trust between the local community of GPs

Those GPs who registered on the online learning network were not highly involved in their local community of GPs. There were also relatively low levels of regular communication, mutual assistance or trust between members. There was no significant difference before and after entering the online network.

Attitudes towards the online network

Prior to entry in the online learning network, participants held positive views towards what they expected to achieve in the network. The largest fears expressed by respondents were issues regarding confidentiality and the sharing of information and ideas. After joining the online network, some participants were less concerned about confidentiality and sharing information and ideas, but others did not receive any information or ideas, and it did not increase the feeling of being in a network.

Website activity

Of the 15 who entered the online learning network, five entered the network for a relatively short period before withdrawing and a further three withdrew after only participating in the initial socialisation activities. The remaining seven members mostly participated until the end of the network. Examination of the patterns of interaction for each topic showed that there was an initial burst of enthusiasm in the online learning network, with many messages being posted and responded. After the first month of the network being operational there was much less interaction and often the interaction would only be between two individuals. In total 141 messages were posted whilst the network was open.

Content analysis of discussion board activity

Participants stated that they hoped to share ideas, learn from each other and get to know other local GPs. This was particularly important for GPs who felt isolated and had difficulties in attending local meetings.

> Hello. I am looking forward to e-meeting other GPs as I work in quite an isolated way. I am hoping to be able to have a place to discuss with and learn from each other.

There were mixed feelings about confidentiality, with half concerned and half having no concerns.

> I must say I don't have any great concerns. I'm just keen to get discussing.

Several participants stated that a benefit of the online learning network was that there was a realisation that they all face the same problems.

> It's been enjoyable reading everyone's messages but I don't think I have learned much about myself. Good to know we all face the same problems.

There was only one small discussion thread in which three participants shared information about physiotherapy referrals. The discussion was superficial with only simple exchange of information with no elaboration or critical discussion.

Telephone interviews (post-evaluation interview)

Four participants were interviewed and each person represented differing levels of engagement in the network, ranging from non-entry to highly participative members. There was no consistent pattern of responses between these groups.

Important reasons for joining the online learning network were curiosity, the need to reduce isolation and to improve computer skills.

> It sounded exciting and sounded like that is where the future would be and I wanted to be part of it.

> I was feeling quite isolated at the time; as a GP I thought it would be a good way to be in touch with GPs in the area.

> Thought it would help me with my electronic skills which are poor really, such as the internet and email.

Two expected the network to provide quick answers to problems.

> What would really have been appreciated was a method of getting quick answers to relatively simple questions.

Common problems that were stated by interviewees included lack of postings by themselves and other network members, lack of clear focus on cooperative learning and not enough time.

> I found it hard to come up with ideas to put onto the network.

> I found it difficult to take seriously because there wasn't much response.

> If people have logged on regularly then we could have got a more meaningful discussions.

> Basically people used it as an excuse to have a bit of a whinge about things they didn't like.

> Don't know how you would be able to practically give me more time.

Suggestions to improve the online network included provision of CPD points, but other members noted that sufficient CPD points were already widely available from other activities, and the need to keep ICT simple.

> I think also the carrot . . . that if you do this then you will get an hour's CME or whatever might have encourage people to have logged on regularly.

> The technical and timing issues are the main things.

Discussion

This case study describes a particular group of GPs within a specific context. The group that was studied was small and the response rate was low. There was a spread of confidence and competence in ICT in the study group, although this was probably higher than the average for GPs in the UK.[10] However, some participants had low levels of ICT skills and this may be a factor in their non-engagement. It also was likely that the online learning network members who did engage were 'early adopters' who already used ICT frequently in their personal and professional lives. However, despite these limitations, the case study reflected the reality of the situation.

Activity within the online learning networks was low. An important aspect of ensuring interaction online is the development of trust and shared understanding between members.[11,12] Low levels of trust and mutual sharing of information were noted by all members before joining the online network and this was not overall significantly increased by participation, despite deliberate online activities to develop this important dimension through online socialisation activities. Trust is developmental and linked to the notion of reciprocity, in which members will tend to only post messages if they feel that other members are contributing.[13] It was noted that there was an initial flurry of online activity but this rapidly tailed off, and a concern for members was the lack of postings.

The use of the online discussions was mainly limited to information exchange rather than an ongoing dialogue with exchange in views. This may be related to the early developmental stage of the online learning network.[7] The level of online discussion is related to the level of trust between members and typically trust increases with the later stages of online network development, resulting in interactive dialogue between members.[7] This active participation in developing new knowledge is essential for learning that is part of CPD.[14]

The difficulties associated with poor engagement in the online learning network have also been noted in other studies of online discussion boards for GPs.[15,16] The aspect of trust has not been identified before for online discussion boards for GPs. Similar difficulties with poor engagement have also been noted in studies of online networks in non-healthcare organisations,[17] and higher education.[18]

The potential of online learning networks is the establishment of an online community of practice in which knowledge is actively created and shared.[19] Much of the literature that promotes the value of online communities of practice as a method to increase organisational performance recognises the importance of active participation rather than simple information exchange.[20] The evaluation of this case study had an objective of identifying the impact on practice following participation in an online structured learning network. No change in practice was noted but this was not surprising since the network did not become established and no active participation occurred.

We recognise that the study group was small but the results reflect the wider difficulties that have been found in studies of online learning networks in non-healthcare and healthcare settings, including GPs outside the UK. We feel that important lessons have been learnt that will be useful to inform further developments and policy decisions for the use of online learning networks for use by GPs for CPD in the UK context.

An important aspect is to ensure high participation and suggestions included an initial (and possibly ongoing) face-to-face meetings for the members of the network and sufficient time allocated to allow members to engage with the online network during their work.[17] We recommend that consideration is given to a wider framework of issues, identical to those that have that has also been suggested as essential for the development of e-learning.[21] The important dimensions are competencies, connectivity and content. Competencies includes the development of skills, not only in the use of ICT, such as basic computer skills, but also how to use discussion boards. It is essential that GPs feel comfortable within an online environment. Connectivity includes the technical aspects of accessing the information through computer systems. The NHSnet may be widespread but there may still be difficulties with interoperability between different systems, including difficulties in access due to NHSnet security features. Content includes the design of the online learning network, to enable it to be easily used to achieve active participation rather than simple information exchange. This may include the provision of online facilitation (often called moderating).[7] It is important to remember that any ICT system has to interface with a human being and that ICT systems should be designed with the user in mind.[22]

Conclusion

Online learning networks offer an exciting opportunity for GPs to share knowledge and learn. These networks have the potential to become a major component for CPD by GPs We have reported a single case study of a pilot project and there is an urgent need to undertake further research to see if our findings are typical of the problems that occur when online learning networks are introduced for CPD by GPs in the UK. However, if our findings are replicated, then the expected potential will not be reached unless the underlying difficulties are considered.

Acknowledgments

We thank the support of NW (the host primary care organisation in north-west England) and the GPs who participated in this study. We have preserved anonymity due to the nature of the findings.

References

1 Parboosingh JT (2002) Physician communities of practice: where learning and practice are inseparable. *Journal of Continuing Education for Health Professionals.* **22**: 230–32.
2 Barab SA, Kling R and Gray JH (2004) *Designing for Virtual Communities in the Service of Learning.* Cambridge University Press, Cambridge.
3 Department of Health (2001) *Working Together – Learning Together: a framework for lifelong learning in the NHS.* Department of Health, London.
4 Horne M, Skidmore P and Holden J (2003) *Learning Communities and NHSU.* National Health Service University, London.
5 Department of Health (1998) *Information for Health: an information strategy for the modern NHS 1998–2005.* Department of Health, London.
6 Broadbent B (2002) *ABCs of e-Learning.* Jossey-Bass/Pfeiffer, San Francisco.

7 Salmon G (2000) *E-moderating: the key to teaching and learning on-line.* Kogan Page, London.
8 Weinstein K (1995) *Action Learning.* HarperCollins, London.
9 Inglis S (1994) *Making the Most of Action Learning.* Gower, London.
10 Wilson SM (1999) Impact of the internet on primary care staff in Glasgow. *Journal of Medical Internet Research.* **1**:1.
11 Walther J (1996) Computer mediated communication: impersonal, interpersonal and hyperpersonal interaction. *Communication Research.* **23**: 3–43.
12 Lesser EL (2000) *Knowledge and Social Capital.* Butterworth-Heinemann, Woburn, MA.
13 Gibson CB and Manuel JA (2003) Building trust. In Gibson CB and Cohen SG (eds). *Virtual Teams That Work.* Jossey-Bass, San Francisco.
14 Jarvis P (1995) *Adult and Continuing Education.* Routledge, London.
15 Fox N (1998) *The WISDOM '97 final report.* ScHARR, Sheffield.
16 Curran VR, Hoekman T, Gullivar W *et al.* (2000) Web-based continuing medical education. (II): Evaluation study of computer-mediated continuing medical education. *Journal of Continuing Education for Health Professionals.* **20**: 106–19.
17 Gibson CB and Cohen SG (2003) *Virtual Teams That Work.* John Wiley, San Francisco, CA.
18 Richardson B and Cooper N (2003) Developing a virtual interdisciplinary research community in higher education. *Journal of Interprofessional Care.* **17**: 173–82.
19 Lesser EL and Storck J (2001) Communities of practice and organizational perform-ance. *IBM Systems Journal.* **40**: 831–41.
20 Cothrel J and Williams RL (1999) On-line communities: helping them form and grow. *Journal of Knowledge Management.* **3**: 54–60.
21 Library and Information Commission (2003) *2020 Vision.* Library and Information Commission, London.
22 Kling R (1999) What is social informatics and why does it matter? *D-Lib Magazine.* **5**:1.

Chapter 16

Developing an effective email discussion group

John Sandars, Richard McDonough, Jennifer McDonough and Jonathan Burton

---

Key points

- Email has the potential to offer an opportunity for collaborative learning between healthcare professionals.
- Email offers an established method to communicate but an important barrier is the new use of an established technology.
- The provision of leadership and structure is important to ensure successful learning.
- An important aspect of the learning is the opportunity to share information and to reflect on the comments before replying to messages.

Introduction

The value of collaborative learning is well established and in primary care this often occurs in the practice setting. There are a variety of opportunities, such as through a formal practice-based learning group, or informally by corridor or coffee room discussions. However, many healthcare professionals find it increasingly difficult to find a convenient time and place to share experiences with colleagues.

Email offers a convenient, simple and reliable method to communicate between individuals.[1] Most people will have access to email, either at work or home, and feel comfortable using the technology. Messages can be sent, received and read at any time. There is always a delay between sending a message and receiving the reply (so-called, asynchronous communication) but sending and receiving can be done in quick succession. There are other methods that use different technologies, such as chat rooms or discussion boards, but most individuals in primary care contexts do not have experience of these methods.

In this chapter we describe the experience of a time-limited email discussion group that was developed between two general practitioners (based in Manchester (JS) and Suffolk (JB)) and a practice nurse and a practice manager (both based in south-west London (JM and RM)).

The email discussion group

The aim was to assess the efficacy of email as a medium for peer discussion of practice-based problems. The method of communication for the group was by ordinary email, with all emails being copied to all group members. One of the group (JS) acted as group leader and sent out email instructions to all group members initially and then at each stage of the group process (*see* Box 16.1 for the instructions).

Box 16.1 Instructions on how to perform an email discussion group

Initial instructions

Remember: The personal details of each patient, for example their name, address or age, should remain private to the patient. All emails that are exchanged should not contain information that could be linked to individual patients. Please ensure that the access to all emails respects the confidentiality of the information.

1 Each person identifies one critical incident – more of a 'Aha' experience. Maybe something read or seen related to professional work. Anything that makes us wake up!
2 Write an email. Describe the incident – in 200 words. State why this incident is being presented. How did it challenge your knowledge/ beliefs? How would you like the rest of the group to help you? Please try to be specific.
3 Post email to all members of the group.
4 Please give and receive comments from other group members. You should reply to each person at least once, but the more the better!

Second instruction

1 State reflection on feedback. What are your thoughts to what has been sent?
2 State new thoughts about the initial incident. What do you think after receiving the comments?

Final instruction

1 What do you think helped in the process of sharing your problem in the group?
   – What did we do collaboratively that we could not have done by ourselves?
   – What difficulties did you encounter? How can they be overcome?
2 What was your overall impression with the use of email as a method of collaboration?
   – What helped?
   – What hindered?
   – What can be done differently next time?

Each member was asked to remember a real-life practice-based problem from his or her own practice work, abbreviate it and then circulate it to the other participants. Group members were each required to set out the help that they actually wanted in resolving their puzzlement over this problem. Fellow group members responded to this request and there was some further discussion via email. Group members then reflected on how much the discussion had helped them and summed up their views of the advantages and disadvantages of the process.

The personal details of each patient, for example their name, address or age, remained private to the patient. They were not shared between the group members at any time during the project and emails that were exchanged did not contain information that could be linked to individual patients. In addition, some details of the cases were modified to strengthen the degree of anonymity.

A sequential log of all the emails sent was created. By reading through this log it was possible to analyse the responses in this learning group.

The tale of the first general practitioner (JS)

I have been concerned over a consultation with the parents of a persistently coughing baby. It was a Sunday morning at the out-of-hours centre and the parents were at the end of their tether, especially as the mother had hardly slept for the previous two nights. They were demanding that something was done. No previous treatment had worked and they wanted it sorted out. The child appeared well and I felt under pressure to prescribe something. I prescribed an antihistamine, which is a sedative medicine. This medicine is not recommended for young children in the *British National Formulary* but has, in practice, quite often been used for children. I want to explore the extent to which care should be dictated by a patient and in what way.

Quickly, there was a series of emails from the other members of the group. They wanted more information about the parents, the child and why the doctor had felt under pressure. Clearly the original story was in need of some clarification, the others needing to ascertain the mood of the consultation in greater detail. JS answered these queries, perhaps a little frustrated that his story hadn't been immediately 'read' by the others. But for him the nub of the problem was the tension about what might help the family here and what was 'correct and according to the rules' of medicine: he had to think hard.

> 'I think my question is about the tension of 'evidence' and the real-life caring situation. I am breaking guidelines! Surely I must be a 'bad professional'.

He found it reassuring to know that the other participants appreciated the very difficult situation he had been in, trying to help the worn-out parents of a not particularly ill baby. It certainly helped to receive the comments from both the practice manager and the practice nurse. As RM said:

'Putting myself in the parents' position, I suppose I would have expected to have walked out with something more than reassurance, i.e. a prescription.'

JS felt that the group had offered him support in what was a tricky situation.

The tale of the practice manager (RM)

A female, registered elsewhere, had requested, by a letter addressed to me, that she be accepted as a patient at the practice. She related that she was not satisfied with the care that she had received at her present practice. She said that she would like to see a lady doctor, and that there were some delicate (but not entirely stated) health matters to discuss. The doctors in my practice discussed the request. However, as there was a practice policy of only registering whole families, and as the patient could not always be guaranteed that she would be able to see a lady doctor, they asked me to write to her and turn down this request. This I did. I thought that this would be the end of the matter, but I received a written reply from her, requesting that the request be reconsidered for three reasons.

1   The policy of only registering family groups did not take into account the barriers that many women in the community face.
2   Many women in our diverse, multicultural and multifaith society will only find a female doctor acceptable.
3   Furthermore, she said she would wait patiently to see the lady doctor.

I have not yet replied but seek advice from the group about whether my original letter had shown evidence of discrimination. I would like group members to say what they might have done.

Each of the other three members of the group responded giving some advice to the practice manager. One GP (JB) thought that the practice had not shown discrimination as it simply stated its reasonable policy about only registering family groups. The other GP (JS) had had similar experiences in practice. The practice nurse (JM) remarked that the patient might have successfully registered if she hadn't written the original letter. There was also a discussion as what was 'reasonable' – who should determine this. Both GPs pointed out that there had to be a balance between the needs of the individual patient and those of the practice. JS felt that rules were essential. The other (JB) felt that the more you stuck to rules, the more you 'collided' with the reality of people's lives.

RM had found that the feedback was only partially helpful. It had not exactly answered his questions and he felt that 'in hindsight, I think I should have asked for more feedback in answer to my original questions.'

The tale of the second general practitioner (JB)

At coffee time today we were discussing the 'falling standards of behaviour in public' and the discussion then went on to the question of unruly children in the consulting room. A mother came today with three boys under the age of 11, the youngest of whom was the patient. The other two climbed on and off the examination couch, pulling down the paper sheet. This was happening behind the mum's back but when I politely asked them to stop doing it she did not comment. Some parents have better behaved and more biddable children than others but unruly kids are far from uncommon. There is a toy box in the room I use, but the toys are only suitable for toddlers. Any thoughts on this problem – what ways can individual practitioners deal with it and would it be appropriate for the practice as a whole to think it through, or do we just have to put up with it?

There was a brisk round of emails suggesting different approaches, and two members of the group agreed that it was almost impossible to concentrate on the problem in hand when other family members were being unruly. The first general practitioner (JS) would consider stopping the consultation and rescheduling it without children. The practice manager (RM) suggested the help of a receptionist to look after the children and the possibility of writing a letter to the parents, after the consultation, as something of a reprimand. The practice nurse (JM) also suggested the help of a receptionist to look after the 'spare' children, but this would not be possible at busy times. She also explained that in her practice they had put locks on low level cupboards for this very reason.

JB reflected on these problems over the next few days and he also shared his thoughts with friends and relatives. He had found that the feedback and consequent personal reflection had clarified his views. Although, personally, he found unruly children difficult to deal with, he realised that harm reduction and trying to keep the peace were his chosen responses to this sort of problem.

There is a variety of opinions, varying from punitive to harm reduction. As I think about it all, I am more and more uncomfortable with any behaviour that raises the temperature in the consulting room.

The tale of the practice nurse

My problem is about two patients who are infected with a blood-borne virus. In both cases they have been happy to admit this but request the diagnosis is not put on to the computer. In the 'old' days one would simply have a system whereby the notes could have a colour code but nowadays this is not possible in a paper-light practice.

My concerns are:

1 Patient rights.
2 Health & Safety.
3 Inadequate medical records.
4 Not knowing what medication they are being prescribed in secondary care.

How do you get round this problem so that the other doctors and nurses in the practice are aware of the diagnoses?

One GP (JS) took the view that there might be, with the patient's consent, some compromises about the completeness of the notes, sections of which could be put into more hidden sections of the computer system. Or, if all else failed, it could be ensured that the patient received all his/her care from hospital and none from the practice. JM was dubious about the latter choice as the practice would still have a patient registered and had a duty to give care. 'Are we allowed to refuse to give care?' she asked. However, RM and one GP (JB) were sure that the full patient history had to be entered onto the computer, whatever the extent of the hospital involvement. Somehow the patient had to be persuaded that this was necessary and helped to see that his/her notes were subject to strict rules of confidentiality. As the practice manager said, 'this just cannot be swept under the carpet with covert messages'. Such action was needed for 'reasons of complete and safe care and to protect staff who might be taking blood'. RM went on to raise the query as to how the practice might accurately complete an insurance report without such full information, but no one took him up on this point.

The learning experience for the group members

The level of interaction was less dynamic, less 'to and fro' than might occur in a conversation with all participants present. All group members reported positively on the learning experience. Everyone found it useful to get a variety of different views from colleagues of differing professional backgrounds working in primary care. This variety and mutuality seems to have been one of the main factors, which made the group a positive learning experience.

> A multi-professional group working in a common area of healthcare –
> all being aware of the culture of GP practices.
>
> (RM)

> The interest generated by these problems shows that there is a
> commonality about dilemmas in healthcare – even when a particular
> problem is unique.
>
> (JB)

> Able to be involved and reflect on other people's problems and not just
> nursing-related problems.
>
> (JM)

Getting feedback and different perspectives.

(JS)

It was also noted that in this particular approach to group learning there was time to reflect between the various stages of the debate.

Having time to think about the responses before replying.

(JM)

Time to reflect and discuss with others outside the group in between the phases of the email collaboration, thereby deepening the reflection process, in a way which is not possible in a live group.

(JB)

However, there was a general feeling that with this approach to group learning each person's individual problems might not be adequately dealt with.

I had no problems with sharing my problem but it appears that as a group we didn't respond fully enough to all the members' requests for help and feedback.

(JB)

As a first time exercise, not knowing the breadth and depth to go with any particular problem, I felt that my particular problem was not adequately dealt with.

(JM)

The difficulties experienced by the group members

Three of the four members found working with email difficult. JB, whilst enjoying the process as a whole, found the email process 'chaotic – it lacked the rhythm of normal human communication', and JM complained that it was 'very difficult and confusing to have so many emails as I am not used to using this method of communication regularly'. RM said that the process was hindered by the need to unscramble 'all the responses chronologically . . . Group members can send more than one email on the same day to more than one problem.' RM suggested that there needed to be a more systematic approach to dealing with the flow of emails.

The confusion in the communication was a serious problem. JM inferred that this very problem made her prefer an alternative approach to discussing problems – one-to-one supervision. JB, however, weighed up the negative side of the communication problems with the positive outcomes 'Nevertheless, and taking the downside into consideration, I was able to gain a learning experience of some importance without leaving my study.'

The above comments highlight the difficulties associated with using a new application of an existing technology, although email was familiar to all of the members. The new method and pace of communication by email required an adjustment to existing patterns of use for email. Members had to quickly develop new ways of giving information and feedback. The technical difficulties were mainly related to the archiving of a stream of email messages. There are simple strategies, such as archiving all messages from the group in a separate folder or replying within the body of a received email so that it gradually contains all the messages that have been received and sent by the members. It is expected that more experienced users of email would be aware of these strategies and that these technical issues would be minimised.

The same three members appreciated the importance of the leadership provided by JS, JB and RM stating that the leadership role was essential, and all three saying it had been helpful.

Conclusion

A time-limited email discussion group can lead to significant learning experiences. The problems produced for discussion were appropriate for a multiprofessional group, and members found the mixed professional input and feedback to be useful. Two members, however, found that the feedback on their problems was incomplete. In comparison with a live discussion group, the 'conversation' was more limited, with much briefer responses in each round of communication, so brief in fact that on occasions points raised were not responded to. However, as the discussion was undertaken over a period of time, members found that having time to reflect between the various stages of the process was particularly useful. On the negative side, members found that the email communication was confusing, with messages coming in at various times, often out of logical sequence. Leadership of the group was important, with each stage of the process being orchestrated by the group leader.

There is a need to adjust to email as a form of 'learning communication'. The use of any new technology requires a 'learning curve' and often this may be initially steep. However, with increasing use there is adaptation, innovation and increased confidence. It is expected that users who have more experience in handling a large variety and number of emails would not have the same technical difficulties.

Once there is a flow of messages they will begin to form an ever-increasing stack. It is important that there is some type of system for storing these messages. The value of web-based discussion boards is that messages can be linked to one another (so-called 'threaded' discussions) but for emails another system has to be developed. There is no ideal system. Suggestions include creating a specific folder in Outlook Express, in which all relevant messages can be archived in date order, or replying to messages by embedding the original message in the text.

This is the first email discussion group for primary care that has been described in the UK. An email discussion group linked to clinical case-discussions has been evaluated in Canadian family physicians and the participants described several advantages over face-to-face groups.[2] Participants found that it provided an opportunity to learn at their own pace and they also valued the time to reflect on the various comments from the group before sending a message. A summary of all the discussions for later review was also noted to be useful.

References

1 Preece J (2000) *Online Communities*. John Wiley and Sons, Chichester.
2 Marshall JN, Stewart M and Ostbye T (2001) Small group CME using e-mail discussions. Can it work? *Canadian Family Physician*. **47**: 557–63.

Chapter 17

Creating a website for your VTS scheme

Nick Foster

Key points

- It is important to initially determine the target group and the purpose of the site.
- A careful step-wise process is essential to ensure that an effective website is produced.
- An important aspect is to keep the format simple.

The start of a good idea

It's a nice badge to wear – 'we have our own website'. It is as if this statement alone that makes a Vocational Training Scheme (VTS) 'up to date' and 'at the cutting edge of technology'. The internet is littered with the empty shells of websites that started off on this basis. However, a website can be used as a successful educational tool and an asset to any VTS. This can be assisted and made easier by following certain rules and that the purpose of this chapter is expounding these rules.

At Nottingham, we started a website about seven years ago. I will immediately put my hands up and admit that our VTS site on the Nottingham VTS (www.nottm-vts.org.uk) is far from perfect. However, from its conception in 1998 I have been through the pain of mistakes, rewritten the site on a major scale at least three times and have accepted that the nirvana of enlightenment will never be reached. But this is a strength and not a weakness.

We now have a dedicated assistant as well as course organiser input into the site to make sure new ideas and innovations can be incorporated within the site. The future site will include online feedback and online assessment. The scheme website has now become integral with our teaching.

The first steps

Determine the target group and the purpose of the site

Appearance and information given on sites varies. I have listed many current VTS sites at the end of this chapter and our website at www.nottm-vts.org.uk/Websites/Medical/VTS.htm for you to make up your own mind. They all give scheme information, some give information about the trainers, the course structure, how to apply and so on. Some are run by postgraduate departments on behalf of VTS schemes, some are run by the VTS itself, perhaps a keen course organiser or trainer. So the first question you should ask yourself is: 'Do I need a website?' Many deaneries hold information on their own Deanery website about VTS schemes. On the whole, the information is rather limited and tends to relate to the organisation of the scheme although deaneries do vary in the amount of information provided.

When designing a website, the first question you need to address is the purpose of the website and how it fits in with your educational aims.

- Who is your target audience?
- What do you want your viewer to get from the site?

Many sites appear to have static information. There are only a handful that are interactive with downloadable educational material, online discussion groups and so on.

Our target groups were the trainers and GP registrars as well as prospective candidates to the scheme. The scheme was large, with 80 GP registrars and 40 trainers. Paper information was huge and often became out of date. Changes to the timetable are inevitable. Posting out papers and teaching material was costly in both time and money.

In 2005, we made the conscious decision to become what has become a fashionable term: 'paperlite'. The educational decision to move from a paper-based scheme to a web-based scheme was in part to force GP registrars and trainers to become computer-literate. All questions are directed to the site. The timetable contains not only the week's topic, but also reading links to be completed before the session. The site is also dynamic as it changes day by day with new information.

Determine roles and responsibilities

The website needs to be managed. You need to decide who will do this. Is it to be done by a sole person, or can others contribute? Think of the website as having four areas of responsibility. These could all be managed by one person, equally they could be managed by a group.

1 **Site strategy:** How will the website fit in the overall running of the scheme? Is the website purely for prospective candidates to the scheme or will it be integrated into the scheme? Are you going to have it password protected or is it open to all?
2 **Editorial strategy:** Who decides what material is put on the site? Is it a sole contributor or are others involved in providing the material? At Nottingham, we encourage lecturers to provide material for GP registrars to read and assimilate before the half-day release by making it available on the website. The course organisers are responsible for getting hold of this material and then forwarding it to the website publisher.
3 **Web management:** How will you know whether the information is getting to the intended audience? We took the radical step of ceasing to provide lecture notes. We felt it was the GP registrars' responsibility to download the material

and print it off as well as to read it (adult-centred learning). In addition, twice a year we ask for feedback on what changes they would like to see on the website as well as course structure.

4 **Content provision:** Ensure the content of the site is current and that it is published or archived in a timely fashion. Last year's exam dates are no good to anyone. Archive or delete them.

Determine how the site is updated

How often you update the site depends on what information you are trying to provide. The more you move to provide interactivity, the bigger demand it will place on your resources. If you do decide to be more 'educational', ask the question: 'How will the updates be managed?'

With one person responsible for the site, this was easy. Web data was uploaded from a single PC to the internet server. Increasing the numbers of contributors has led us to change this method of updating. We now update the website directly on the server. This means it can be updated any where at any time.

One of my pet hates is to visit a website and see the last time anything was added to the site was two or more years ago. Do you hold any value or credence to the information on the site if the last time anyone touched it was two years ago?

Whatever approach you decide to follow, be it solely information or the move into an educationally interactive site, there are steps you can follow to make the site a pleasure to browse and use.

Website creation

Do-it-yourself or get someone to do it for you?

There are three options open to you when making the decision to move into the area of web creation and design:

1 build your own site and maintain everything yourself
2 hire a web professional to handle everything for you
3 a middle-ground: hiring a web professional to set up the site and then maintain parts or all of it yourself.

The first option could face you with lacking the skill and experience to do it right, while the second option may leave you feeling powerless to manage your own site. The third option is a halfway house.

Box 17.1 Easy website creation

Tip

Website creation has moved on over the last 3 years and it is now possible to produce a good-looking, quick and easy website using products such as Microsoft FrontPage® (www.microsoft.com) or Macromedia Dream-weaver® (www.macromedia.com).

Creating a website is an ongoing process. It is not static or a one-off, it has to be kept up to date and updated on a regular basis. There are plenty of web design companies around who can be paid to do this. However, you will still have to write some of the copy, discuss the structure and layout of the site. It may therefore pay you to think about creating a website yourself. This will have the following advantages:

- It is far cheaper.
- You have total control about the layout of the site.
- You can update it as often as you wish.

There are some disadvantages of course. Creating online questionnaires and database entries takes skill and may be beyond your immediate capabilities. The use of animations, flashy graphics and so on may require a good grasp of web coding language such as HTML.

In the rush to have the 'coolest' site design, you can forget who you are designing the site for: the target audience. Your audience might find that Flash movie on the first page irritating after viewing it multiple times. There are pitfalls you should be aware of when creating your site. I will try and highlight useful functions to include in your design and steer you away from what can only be described as 'bad' ideas.

A good example of a 'bad' idea was the early use of frames on websites. The concept sounds good – frames split the page into two or more sections, which the browser identifies separately. Unfortunately some browsers cannot interpret a site with frames properly because they read 'down' each frame, rather than across the frameset. A better design is to use a 'shared border' which although it sounds similar is in fact quite different. Borders can be shared between many pages giving it that unified appearance without the mess frames imposed.

Another example of a 'bad idea' is the page marked 'under construction' on a live site. This is usually associated with an animated cartoon of somebody digging. Not only is this annoying for users, it undermines the professionalism of the site.

Purchasing your website server and domain name.

Buying a domain name is not costly. Registration domains such as .com can be expensive whereas .org.uk is cheaper. Nominet www.nominet.org.uk is the authoritative database of .uk domain name registrations and on this site there are links to many registration agents. You can get deals for as little as £25 giving you a package of 50 email addresses, 4GB of web space, and 2 years' domain name registration.

Box 17.2 Questions to ask when choosing a hosting service

Tip

Make sure the web hosting site server can take the current version of web software you are using. For example, the latest Microsoft FrontPage® server extensions may not be loaded by your web host.

Choosing your web package

This boils down to personal preference. Personally I have used Microsoft FrontPage for many years. Consider purchasing a 'Teach yourself' book on your chosen package. This will allow you to fully understand how the package works. This spurred me into setting up an intranet website within our practice to store practice documents and also our own practice website using the same software.

Another popular product is Macromedia Dreamweaver®, which has the added benefit of providing a suite of other integrated software linking into their main product – but at a price.

At the other extreme you could just learn the HTML language and write the pages yourself. Although some would consider this the purist approach, it will take a considerable time to get to anywhere near producing such layouts as the GUI (graphical user interface) applications of FrontPage or Dreamweaver. But help is at hand if you do wish to see the HTML language behind your webpage

Using FrontPage one can change font size, colour, position, insert pictures and insert tables very easily. In addition, FrontPage (along with most web editing software) also has the option of seeing the HTML coding behind the page. This has two immediate benefits:

1 It allows you to easily debug problems that can appear on your webpage. Most commonly these are unlinked hyperlinks that do not appear on the document's layout page. These can be spotted in HTML.
2 There are components you may wish to insert that do not come with FrontPage such as text showing date and time on your website. By using Java applets (short pieces of code that run under Java), you can cut and paste these applets into your web page. There are many websites that provide access to free Java applets for you to use (www.bravenet.com/, http://javascriptkit. com).

Thinking about your design

Don't leap into building a website before you understand what you want to accomplish. The more carefully you plan, the better off you will be when you begin to build your site. The best way to get ideas is to look at other websites and use their design and structure as a basis to start from.

Have a look at our scheme website at www.nottm-vts.org.uk.

Note the virtual white background, the absence of a long scrolling page that goes on and on, basic clear readable text, a clear menu, last modified date, a few pictures to give colour to the page but not to dominate it. The moving text of 'Program Changes' draws the eye to the important information I want the GP registrars and trainers to see. By the end of this chapter you will be able to critique a site, noting good and bad points.

The fundamentals of good web design

Understanding the language

The original language of the web was HTML (hypertext markup language). The benefit of a common language is the ability for browsers of whatever type to be able to read web pages on the internet. There were limitations with HTML and therefore over time the language has been altered. The ability of a browser viewing a website therefore depends on how up-to-date their web browsing software is.

XML (Extensible Markup Language) is the next-generation HTML: it enables systems to exchange data more easily and is more useful for database applications, for example allowing users to access and update the own records and personalised information according to user preference and so on. Unfortunately there is no backward compatibility between XML and HTML and therefore users with older browsers would be excluded if you published exclusively in XML.

This has been addressed by the creation of XHTML (eXtensible HyperText Markup Language). XHTML reformats HTML as an XML application, overcoming the problem of backward compatibility. There are software tools available to allow one to convert old HTML documents to the newer XHTML.

A second innovation has been the creation of cascading style sheets (CSS). This allows one to separate styling elements from the content and structure of web pages, allowing pages to be structured and styled consistently and enabling content to be loaded quickly. Again, older browsers may have difficulty implementing some CSS code.

A third type of innovation are active server pages (ASP). ASP files produce ordinary HTML and work with any browser but they do need a Windows NT server to run programs written using a combination of HTML, JavaScript and VBScript. These files can be recognised as they carry an ASP suffix. The great thing about ASP files is that they enable the ability to integrate databases within the website. Scripting languages such as PHP and Perl provide similar functionality for non-Windows servers.

If you do wish to use these facilities, it is important to make sure your hosting service supports them. At Nottingham, we had to move service providers as, although our original supplier allowed us to use FrontPage, it did not have the FrontPage Server Extensions enabling us to use ASP files and hence we were unable to use the database functionality within FrontPage.

In an unregulated world, there has been an attempt to provide some uniformity as to how the web should be structured, its coding language and so on. Called the World Wide Web Consortium or W3C (www.w3.org), it currently recommends XHTML 1.0 as the mark-up language to be used together with Cascading Style Sheets 2. This is important to understand as some users may have older browsing software and therefore may have difficulty reading your site.

Should all pages be in HTML?

HTML is not always the most suitable language for publishing information on the web. Large documents, the presence of columns and lots of graphics, detailed tabular information, are all better published in a print-ready format such as

Adobe Acrobat Portable Document Format (PDF), Rich Text Format (RTF) or simply as plain text or a Microsoft Word document, which has become an international standard.

Adobe Acrobat has produced the Portable Document Format (PDF) as an industry standard. The advantage of this format is that it can be read on any machine using any operating system such as Apple Mac, Microsoft Windows or UNIX. Users do need Adobe Acrobat Reader to access PDF files. Although in order to produce PDF files you have to buy the appropriate software, the reading software (Adobe Acrobat Reader) is provided free. For those users without the software, it is useful to have a link to Adobe in order for the reader to be downloaded free of charge (www.adobe.com/products/acrobat).

An alternative is Microsoft Word and, again, a free viewer from Microsoft enables a person without Microsoft Word installed on the computer to read your Microsoft Word document (www.microsoft.com/office/000/viewers.asp).

Many lectures are delivered as PowerPoint presentations these days, and again there are free viewers to enable those users without PowerPoint to be able to view these presentations (www.microsoft.com/downloads/).

Have an easy-to-update design/structure

Just a few years ago many websites had spinning globes, animated construction workers and many other cartoon graphics. Whilst appearing very pretty, they added little. Your aim should be able to freely add and remove elements from your pages with little or no trouble.

Aim to have fast-loading pages. This is one of the oldest rules in the book. Be aware that your target audience may not all have broadband. Not all users will be using Internet Explorer. Netscape Navigator, Opera and Mozilla Firefox are other web browsers that are used. Be aware that download speeds vary. The last few years of web experience have shown that if people have to wait more than 10 seconds to see your page then they will lose interest. Just because your broadband connection only takes 5 seconds to download a page, don't forget that it could take 30 seconds for a user who is connected at a slower speed.

Box 17.3 Hot tips for an effective website

Tip

- Your homepage file size should not exceed 40KB and should load within 5 seconds.
- Your other page file size should not exceed 120KB and should load within 20 seconds.
- Document files should not exceed 300KB. Advise the user of the file size in advance.
- The better the HTML construction, the less time it will take for the page to load.

Images

The heaviest aspects of most web pages are pictures. Concentrate on making images as light as possible without making them look too ugly. This is commonly referred to as 'optimisation'. Many programs like Adobe Photoshop, Macromedia Fireworks and Paint Shop Pro have the built-in capability to create images that are as light as possible. These are called 'web-optimised images'. Because the majority of web browsers recognise GIF (Graphic Interchange Format) and JPEG (Joint Photographics Experts Group) images, these two formats are used most often for saving web images. Images that use a limited palette should be GIFs and should be generated using the web palette.

Some computers are only capable of displaying up to 256 colours. If you reduce the colour depth of the image to 8 bits (256 colours) before placing it on your web page, its appearance will be more consistent. File size affects the majority of users accessing a web page. As the size of an image file increases, it takes more time to download, so viewers have a longer wait. Use a file format that reduces the image size most efficiently while keeping the quality as high as possible. A single image should not be larger than 30kb. If you use larger images, warn the user and display the file size – use a thumbnail image for preference. Don't use large images on the homepage.

If you are tempted to use an animated GIF file, do not let it exceed 30kb. They should cycle no more than four times before stopping.

If you use a small font on an image, avoid blurring the text by switching off the anti-aliasing.

Use the templates in your web package

Use page templates for your website. It's far easier to add new pages if you can start from a page that already has the basic navigation and site graphics in place built into a template. Macromedia Dreamweaver and Microsoft FrontPage offer useful templates and standard reusable libraries of site graphics and HTML that make it easy to create new pages and maintain your site. This will enable you to have a sense of uniformity throughout your site. Templates are designed to combine the best combinations of colours and fonts.

Your website should be easy to read

1 Choose your text and background colours carefully. Avoid backgrounds that obscure text or font colours that are hard to read.

Look for high contrast using single solid background colours. The best example comes from using the two colours black and white. Another good colour combination is light yellow and dark blue. Text should always be a contrasting colour to the background to avoid any blurring on screen. Pale text on a dark background will be difficult to read.

Avoid using red and green together as this will cause problems for colour-blind users. Similarly, avoid colour combinations that cause difficulties, including red and purple, yellow and white/light grey, pastel pink and lavender.

2 The most legible fonts are the standard serif (usually Times) and sans-serif

(usually Arial or Helvetica) ones. Avoid decorative or cursive fonts such as Brush Script.

Be careful choosing font style. Italicised, oblique or condensed fonts are more difficult to read than standard typefaces. Text in CAPITALS and **Bold** tends to stand out and 'shout' at the reader. Similarly, text that is underlined is best avoided as this usually indicates that the text is hyperlinked.

3 Text should be short and concise. Make your text easier to understand by following these points:
   – Because the screen layout is designed going from top to bottom, summarise the key points in the first paragraph.
   – Make sure you try and put the most important point first and the rest in descending order of importance.
   – You will be tempted to fill the page up with text. Be ruthless with the words that you use, cut text down to at least 50% shorter than you would normally use in a written document.
   – Try to show some structure on the page by breaking up the text with clear headings and subheadings.
   – Using bullet points in a list is shorter and neater.
   – Make sure that each page can be read in isolation.

4 Avoid graphic images as backgrounds. Graphic images as backgrounds can make a website more aesthetically pleasing, but can make your website more difficult to read. It may look nice to have the watermark crest of some organisation appearing very faintly as the background to your page, but it is very irritating as often the watermark sits behind text and distracts from the page.

5 Use links. One of the great features of the web is the ability to have links to other documents and other sites. Links can enrich the content of any website and users find them valuable, especially when set in context. It is helpful to have the links on the page itself rather on a separate 'useful links' page.

Think about where you put your link. It can be distracting in the middle of documents and therefore some people recommend that links appear after the text which they relate to. Make the link relevant to the text it follows and make sure that they are easily recognisable. The standard convention of highlighting them in blue and underlining them should be reserved for this style of linkage. It is therefore a good idea to avoid underlining any text as this may be considered a link.

Ensuring links go to the expected page is covered later in this chapter.

6 The basic elements of your page should all be in place:
   (a) An informative title with the creator's identity or institution with a creation or revision date. The revision date will indicate to the user how up-to-date the website is.
   (b) At least one link to a local home page or menu page with the 'home page' URL (Uniform Resource Locator) on the major menu pages of your site. When planning the homepage, make sure that users don't need to know the filename of the homepage to find it. This facility is automatically built in to software packages like Microsoft FrontPage, where the web page index.htm is automatically assigned as the homepage of the site. If you entered www.nottm-vts.org.uk you would be automatically directed to www.nottm-vts.org.uk/index.htm. The homepage is very important and

should be clearly accessible from each page of your site. Ensure that the main navigation menu is on the homepage and that the main sections of the website are only one click from the homepage. Imagine that the homepage is your calling card; you would want to make sure that the organisation name, logo and contact details are all present.

(c) A major crime committed by many web designers is the lack of good navigation and good menu structure. Users should always be able to return easily to your home page and to other major navigation points in the site. These basic links should be present and in consistent locations on every page. Graphic buttons will provide basic navigation links and create a graphic identity that tells users they are within the site domain. Button bars are also the most logical place for links back to your home page or to other menu pages related to the current page. Links to documents should be in a new window so that when closed, the user is taken back to the original URL. All to often the user can get lost within the site, unable to get back, having opened a document that when closed also closes the web browser. How easy is it for someone to get around your website? In other words, how usable is it? If someone has to 'hunt' for your 'home' link or your contact information, then you have a usability problem. Menus should generally be in HTML. The scripts that trigger drop-down menus can cause problems for users with screen readers and screen magnifiers.

(d) Try to avoid pop-up windows. Pop-up windows do not work on all browsers and if they are triggered by JavaScript, they will need a <noscript> alternative. Another problem with pop-up windows is that they can be seen as advertising windows and therefore be blocked by anti-spyware software installed to prevent pop-up windows occurring. Spyware is becoming more of a problem and many internet security software utilities such as Norton will see a pop-up window as a threat and block it.

(e) A well-organised table of contents can be a major navigation tool in your website. The table is more than a list of links – it gives the user an overview of the organisation, extent and narrative flow of your site.

Organise the information you wish to deliver in a logical way

There are five basic steps in organising your information:

Box 17.4 Organising the information

1 Divide your content into logical units.
2 Establish a hierarchy of importance among the units.
3 Build a site that closely follows your information structure.
4 Information flow, a website is not the same as a book or a magazine.
5 Concise chunks of information are better suited to the computer screen.

---

1 **Divide your content into logical units:** Avoid confusing web pages containing mixed information. Try and break the information down into logical units and display these appropriately. Elements within our website include:

   - Timetable, List of Trainers, GP registrars, and Course Organisers as well as the various groups they are in
   - Courses for GP registrars to attend as well as important exam dates
   - Educational syllabus and methods of assessment
   - Summative assessment
   - PMETB regulations regarding training
   - Trainer and GP registrar information
   - The MRCGP exam
   - A Scheme prospectus for those wishing to apply to Nottingham
   - Out of Hours regulations and structure
   - How to email the scheme.

2 **Establish a hierarchy of importance among the units:** Because our scheme is a paper-light scheme, all the information is found on the website. Our timetable is very important so it appears at the top of the list on the home page.

   On the other hand, emailing the scheme, although to be encouraged, is less important and therefore appears lower down in the menu.

3 **Build a site that closely follows your information structure:** When we changed from a paper-based scheme to a web-based scheme, we had to critically appraise our current hard copy information. We found our original information unstructured and confusing. There were numerous assessment forms and documents, confusing to us as course organisers, let alone the trainers and GP registrars.

   Use the opportunity to reassess this information. Unfortunately, some sites have transferred the ongoing text-based confusion and therefore the website appears confusing and disorganised.

4 **A website is not the same as a book or a magazine:** A book consists of chapters and a page structure that is designed to be linear. You start at page 1 and move through the book until you get to the end. You may wish to look at a specific chapter, but relevant information appearing in another chapter will not be available to you until you reach that chapter. A website, on the other hand, is nonlinear – there are no chapters, instead there are connected threads or hyperlinks. Do not base your website on a book structure. Instead consider it as menus and linked items.

5 **Concise chunks of information are better suited to the computer screen:** The screen limits the view of long documents. Long web pages tend to disorient readers; they require users to scroll long distances and to remember what is off-screen. Keep each page simple.

Checking website links and accessibility

Make your website appear in search engines

When you are searching for something on the internet, you will properly use your favourite search engine and type in a few keywords. You will then probably select the first page in the list that looks as if it will give you the information that you want. The position of each entry depends on its ranking by the search engine you have chosen. Search engines generally look at the placement of keywords in the web title page, keywords meta tag, text on the page and description meta tags.

Each search engine analyses the location of keywords and evaluates or ranks a web page differently. However, there are general tips that you can use to get a more favourable search engine ranking for your web page.

A meta tag is a special Hypertext Markup Language (HTML) tag that provides information about your web page and is not visible to visitors. Meta tags provide information such as what the page is about (description tag), and which keywords describe the content of the page (keywords tag).

Think of a description that summarises the content on your website. Each search engine has a different limit for the number of characters from a description that is displayed in the search results. These range generally from 150 to 395 characters, so limit your description accordingly.

First, make sure the 'Title' of your HTML document is descriptive. It should stand on its own. The title of our website is the 'Nottingham Vocational Training Scheme'.

The second element is to think of the keywords people would type in to find your site and make sure that they are included near the top of your web page using the correct HTML meta code. The keywords I use on our website include the following: University, Nottingham, education, teaching, vts, vocational, training, scheme, Nottinghamshire, GPR, GP registrar, UK, VTS, Trainee, General Practice, United Kingdom.

The third element is to think of a description for the site. The description given to our site is: 'The Nottingham Vocational Training Scheme for UK General Medical Practice'

Most of the major search engines, such as MSN, Yahoo! and Google, provide links to their registration pages. To find a listing of search engine companies, visit the Search Engine Watch website at http://searchenginewatch.com.

Website links

Having spent many hours creating your website, the last thing you want is for pages to be inaccessible. This may be due to:

- website links to nonexistent pages
- poor accessibility to pages by badly written code.

Pages on the internet are called URLs. A URL (Uniform Resource Locator) is a unique address for a file on the internet. The URL for our home page is www.nottm-vts.org.uk/index.htm. Every other page on our website will have a unique URL. In addition, pictures and documents will all have their specific URL.

Given that URLs are used so frequently, it's important to understand that there are two kinds of URLs: absolute URLs and relative URLs.

An example of an absolute URL is 'www.nottm-vts.org.uk/index.htm', whereas '../index.htm' is an example of a relative URL. The URL '../index.htm' is relative because it relates to the original website address of www.nottm-vts.org.uk.

The irritating nonexistent page is usually due to a broken hyperlink. Broken hyperlinks are links that don't go anywhere. They are often caused by removing a page or by changing the location of a page. They can also be caused by mistyping the page or file name in either the hyperlink or the URL.

Broken hyperlinks can be detected in a number of ways.

- The software package you are using to create your website will almost certainly have a reports page which will cover broken links, both internal links within your website and external links to other websites.
- There are a plethora of companies that for a fee will check your website for broken links and problems.
- Finally there are free website checkers and one of the best is Xenu's Link Sleuth at http://home.snafu.de/tilman/xenulink.html. I use Xenu on a regular basis to check my website for broken links.

Accessibility

If we all just used one browser, life would be easy. Unfortunately there are numerous different browsers and within each browser there are different versions.

There are a range of tools you can use to check the integrity of your website with regards to accessibility, many of these can be used free of charge. World Wide Web Consortium (W3C) www.w3.org/WAI is the agreed international standard and tries to maintain uniformity. These tools will check your site against agreed standards. When I first used these tools I was horrified by the number of errors that were reported. Unfortunately in order to correct these errors you have to be able to edit the mark-up language code – for example HTML – directly and much of this is beyond the novice.

- The W3C automated validator, http://validator.w3.org, is a W3C Markup Validation Service, a free service that checks web documents in formats like HTML and XHTML for conformance to W3C recommendations and other standards.
- The W3C CSS Validation Service at http://jigsaw.w3.org/css-validator/ checks Cascading Style Sheets (CSS) in (X)HTML documents for conformance to W3C recommendations.
- WebXACT is a free online service that lets you test single pages of web content for quality, accessibility and privacy issues and can be found at http://webxact.watchfire.com. It compares sites and individual pages against the W3C guidelines, highlighting areas of concern, together with suggestions for rectifying them.
- 'A-Prompt' can be used to check web page accessibility to people with disabilities. The A-Prompt software tool www.aprompt.ca examines web pages for barriers to accessibility, performs automatic repairs when possible, and assists in manual repairs when necessary.

The NHS identity

The NHS has produced guidelines on how to set out the design, style and technical standards for NHS websites (www.nhsidentity.nhs.uk/websites/index.htm).

I would recommend looking at the site as there is a whole host of information directed not only at maintaining an NHS identity but also advice on website creation.

The NHS is keen that all NHS websites should conform to the NHS identity of professionalism and clarity although much of the guidance is directed towards the public face of the NHS. Nevertheless, despite the fact that the website is primarily intended for professional information, by being in the public domain, the general public will have access to the site.

There are specific requirements for the NHS logo such as colour and the exclusion zone around it, as well as its placement on the page. Whether this is applicable to VTS schemes is currently unclear, as is the requirement to use the nhs.uk web address.

Legal issues

You may wish to consider making a statement with regard to how your website is run covering the management policies and procedures. This could include statements on:

- **Use of the website:** This should state that there is legal relationship between the viewer of the site and yourselves and that if they are not happy with this understanding, then they should not use the site.
- **Intellectual property:** You may wish to make a statement to the effect that you make no guarantee regarding the accuracy, completeness or reliability of any of the content found on the site. For example, the fact that the dates for the MRCGP examination do not appear on your scheme site cannot be held as a reason for the GP registrar failing to register for the exam in time.

  The material written on the site is the property of the site and can be used for personal or non-commercial use. This will stop someone copying your site and publishing it for material gain but should allow someone to download or copy information useful to them and used by them.
- **Links policy:** Although links are provided, you should state that you are not responsible for the views or content of these linked pages neither can you guarantee that these links will work all of the time.
- **Virus protection:** You should state that you cannot guarantee that the site is free from virus code and that users are responsible for making sure that all material is checked for virus code.
- **Copyright:** Copyright is an intellectual property right and in the UK automatically applies to original work. Copyright does not protect ideas or facts, just the presentation. If another person writes your website, make sure you have the copyright assigned to you as part of the contract. This is not such an issue if you write the material for your own site. If you do publish photographs, then it is wise to get permission for those photographs to be published on the internet.

VTS websites

There is an updated list on our own website at www.nottm-vts.org.uk/Websites/Medical/VTS.htm. Feel free to browse!

Chapter 18

Introducing e-learning into an organisation

John Sandars

Key points

- Expect difficulties when e-learning is introduced into any organisation.
- Initial assessment of the organisational readiness for e-learning is essential for success.
- e-learning champions are important agents for organisational change.
- Action research is a useful method for organisational change when technology is introduced.

Introduction

e-learning is something new for most organisations within healthcare – irrespective of their size. Careful planning of the process of introducing e-learning into an organisation is essential if costly mistakes are to be avoided. The general principles are the same whether the organisation is a practice, a vocational training scheme, a primary care organisation or a Deanery. The same general principles also apply across the range of possible e-learning products, whether it is a single CD-ROM or a major web-based programme. An initial assessment will identify key areas for development in the organisation, learning needs of individuals in the organisation and a clear awareness of the associated risks.

Organisational readiness for e-learning

This can be defined as 'the mental or physical preparedness of an organisation for some e-learning experience or action'.[1] The assessment process should consider seven essential components:

1 **Business readiness:** This refers to the priorities of the organisation and requires a consideration of the fundamental question 'Why is e-learning being introduced?' This might appear to be a simple question but it is important to be clear since this will inform all strategic actions. e-learning is new and novel but that is not sufficient reason to embark upon an organisational e-learning venture. There should be a clear and tangible benefit for both the organisation and the members of that organisation.

2 **Technology readiness:** An appropriate technology infrastructure is one of the

critical components in very e-learning venture. First, there has to be the opportunity to access the required technology, such as a computer or internet, and a consideration of where the technology will be accesses is essential. It maybe easy to access broadband at the place of work but not at home. Second, there has to be a technology infrastructure. It is essential that the inevitable faults that occur with all technology can be quickly and easily rectified.

3 **Content readiness:** e-learning content is becoming increasingly available but may not meet the learning needs of the intended audience. A useful analogy is the recommendation of a core textbook for a particular course. It may suit some people but not others. Unfortunately at the moment there is not such a large variety of e-learning materials as there are in print.

4 **Training process readiness:** This refers to the ability of an organisation to analyse, implement and evaluate its use of e-learning to deliver a particular learning opportunity. For example, if a vocational training scheme wished to consider the use of e-learning to deliver educational content related to ophthalmology then there are several approaches. A short web-based presentation could be offered to a whole group, or individual study could be supported by a series of web links to excellent resources or by using a CD-ROM. The decision will depend on the preferences of both the learner and the course organiser.

5 **Culture readiness:** Undoubtedly the success of introducing any e-learning approach will depend on the individual and collective beliefs about e-learning that are held by everyone who is involved. One doubter can influence the whole group.

6 **Human resources readiness:** It is fine to have the right e-learning materials and the technology to use it but the learner has to have the confidence and competence to use the technology. The level of required computer skills is usually not high but many learners find that there is a steep learning curve in their adaptation to e-learning methods.

7 **Financial readiness:** There is the requirement to have adequate funding to pay for the necessary e-learning materials and the technology infrastructure. It is important to remember that many e-learning projects have relied on short-term funding. This has allowed the often initially high financial costs to be overcome but neglect the continuing costs to support advanced technology.

e-learning champion

The literature on introducing change in any organisation highlights the importance of identifying a so-called change agent. This person is usually charismatic, respected within the organisation and most importantly enthusiastic about the need for change. This situation is no different when planning to introduce e-learning.[2]

Action research and organisational change

The origins of action research are in the implementation of change in social systems, when the outcomes of the change were uncertain. For many interventions applied to complex social systems, such as organisations, problems cannot be easily anticipated. Change will occur but it is unknown in what direction!

Action research is a cyclical process in which there is an initial collection of data to ascertain the present situation, an intervention is introduced and then the change is evaluated. The learning and insights from this first cycle are then used to modify the intervention and the second cycle begins. This approach has been used extensively for the implementation of information technology systems.[3]

The strength of action research is that a systematic process to collecting data and applying an intervention is used. Many e-learning interventions are not evaluated and this has implications for funding of short-term projects.

Conclusion

Most e-learning interventions are costly both in financial terms and in the time required to become acquainted with the new technology. Awareness of the potential problems can help to minimise difficulties. Success cannot be guaranteed but the chances of success are higher!

References

1 Haney D (2002) Assessing organizational readiness for E learning. *Performance Improvement.* **41**: 216–221.
2 Broadbent B (2002) *ABCs of e-Learning.* Jossey-Bass/Pfeiffer, San Francisco.
3 Lau F (2004) A review on the use of action research in information systems studies. In Lee A, Liebenau J, DeGross J (eds) *Information Systems and Qualitative Research.* Chapman & Hall, London.

Further reading

An excellent resource on organisational change.

Iles V and Sutherland K (2001) *Organisational Change: A review of healthcare managers, professionals and researchers.* www.sdo.lshtm.ac.uk/publications.htm

Chapter 19

Future trends in e-learning

Alex Jamieson

Key points

- Computer systems will become increasingly ubiquitous and invisible.
- Virtual Learning Environments (VLEs) will become Personalised Learning Environments (PLEs).
- To enhance learning educational media will need to be discursive, adaptive, interactive and reflective.
- The development of the Educational Semantic Web will be aided by increased global storage capacity, the actions of intelligent agents to augment learning and information retrieval, and the capacity of the internet to support, extend and expand human communications capabilities.

Introduction

We are all e-learners now, whether we know it or not. Computing has become such an omnipresent feature of our personal and professional lives in the developed world, it has become part of our 'practice' in so many contexts, that its influence is unavoidable and undeniable. In short, many of us are dependent on computers and the internet in the way we run our lives.

In an article in the *Guardian* of 6 December 2004 the author reported on the results of an 'Internet Deprivation Study' conducted jointly by Yahoo! and 'media communications specialists' OMD (www.omd.com). The study revealed that, in the 1000 households in the USA which were targeted, volunteers for two weeks of 'weblessness' were exceedingly hard to recruit. So many daily activities had become dependent on a web connection that . . .

> All participants in the qualitative portion of the study found living without the Internet more difficult than they expected, and in some cases impossible, because the tools and services the Internet offers were firmly ingrained in their daily lives.

and . . .

> Regardless of age, household income or ethnic background, all participants in the ethnographic research study experienced withdrawal and feelings of loss, frustration and disconnectedness when cut off from the online world. Users described their time offline as

> 'feeling left out of the loop,' having to 'resist temptation' and missing their 'private escape time' during the day.

In addition . . .

> a complementary quantitative study . . . showed the Internet as the communications and research medium of choice. In the quantitative portion, 48 percent of . . . study respondents indicated they could not go without the Internet for more than two weeks.

It is worth noting that while the above might indicate handicapping levels of addictive behaviour, the study reported that . . .

> the Internet affords people the ability to overcome time and distance and to manage communications with a larger social circle, thereby creating an effortless community.

This enhancement of sociability has been reported elsewhere as a positive feature of online communications.[1] We already know that we can, for instance, become part of an online community in the context of our professional learning, and the popularity of some of the best known web-based learning resources for health professionals depends and thrives on user involvement.

Computer hardware and software is developing, however, in ways which will widen the potential for computers to enhance our learning. In this chapter I will briefly examine those developments and the influence they could have on our own e-learning.

Hardware developments and ubiquitous computing

Computers are everywhere, and in many areas of life day-to-day interaction with computer systems can take place without our ongoing awareness of the relationship, let alone its detail and complexity. Anyone with a 'Nectar' card, or similar loyalty card, has their spending behaviour closely monitored and their profile classified into a targetable population grouping. A traveller on the London public transport system with an 'Oyster' card has their detailed movements logged and recorded. In some retail stores, originally in Japan, owners of store loyalty cards or of purchased products with embedded Radio Frequency Identification tags (RFID tags or 'arphids') are identified when they enter the store, are tracked within it, and could potentially be tracked after they leave. In the UK large supermarkets now use this technology to track tagged items through the supply chain, and to aid with security. A hospital in Japan is using arphid rings instead of patient identity tags to link patients to their records. 'Smart dust' is the name given to tiny processors with built-in transmitters, each not much larger than a grain of sand. They can be configured to create a mobile wireless network wherever they are, and could be scattered over machinery to monitor movement, or over people such as the attendees at a conference for the same purpose. There are countless other possible applications.

These fledgling phenomena of the era of 'ubiquitous computing' are realisations of the world predicted by Mark Weiser of the Xerox Palo Alto Research Centre (PARC) in a highly influential article in *Scientific American* in 1991, entitled 'The Computer for the 21st Century',[2] in which he states:

> The most profound technologies are those that disappear. They weave themselves into the fabric of everyday life until they are indistinguishable from it.

He continues with an example of a technological development already embedded in our culture,

> Consider writing, perhaps the first information technology: the ability to capture a symbolic representation of spoken language for long-term storage freed information from the limits of individual memory. Today this technology is ubiquitous in industrialised countries. Not only do books, magazines and newspapers convey written information, but so do street signs, billboards, shop signs and even graffiti. Candy wrappers are covered in writing. The constant background presence of these products of 'literacy technology' does not require active attention, but the information to be conveyed is ready for use at a glance. It is difficult to imagine modern life otherwise.

He gives the more recent example of the electric motor as a technology which has all but disappeared in, say, the motor car, which in modern versions can easily have more than 20 electric motors fulfilling all kinds of functions, but very much in the background. The 'disappearance' of such technological innovation, in Weiser's argument, is the consequence of human psychology and not of the technology itself. Once we become familiar with something we cease to be so consciously aware of it.

Weiser argues that the idea of ubiquitous computing runs counter to current trends of mobile and multimedia computing which focus us on the machine itself, or of 'virtual reality' which simulates the world rather than enhancing it. He uses the term 'embodied virtuality' to signify the contrast:

> . . . the process of drawing computers out of their electronic shells. The 'virtuality' of computer-readable data – all the different ways in which it can be altered, processed and analysed – is brought into the physical world.

In the world of embodied virtuality there may be hundreds of computers in a room, in all shapes and sizes and degrees of invisibility. Already there are computers in items of domestic electronic equipment which help to activate the world. These machines and more will be interconnected in a ubiquitous network. In particular, focusing on devices that transmit and display information more directly than the above, there are two issues of crucial importance: location and scale.

Computers in embodied virtuality will be aware of where they are (e.g. at home, or in the workplace), and will adapt their behaviour accordingly. They will come in myriad shapes and sizes and will perform different discrete tasks. In Weiser's imagined world it could be that 'tabs' will replace Post-It® notes and be incorporated into ID cards, 'pads' will replace A4 notepads and 'boards' will replace blackboards/flip charts/white boards.

Buildings will know who is inside and where they are from the tabs they wear. Work will return to a real desktop and people will be able to arrange their work on tabs and pads instead of cluttering their PC screens with icons. Pads with their inbuilt processors could be throwaway so that they can be picked up and used anywhere and have no individual identity or importance, just like sheets of paper now. They will link to the user just by being used, and data will be recorded centrally via the tab the user is wearing in their ID badge.

A board-sized computer can clearly function as a large display screen, but might also serve as an electronic bookcase from which documents could be downloaded onto a tab or pad. This could ultimately emulate the ease of use of books themselves but could be accessible to large numbers of people simultaneously. Board displays could be open in more than one location and could be 'shared' by people in different rooms any distance apart. The actual information displayed on a board could be decided by the software and tailored to the user automatically. The 'interactive whiteboard' now commonly used in schools and elsewhere is an early manifestation of some of these ideas. It is worth remembering that it essentially embodies technology which was available 15 years ago.

The real power of the concept of ubiquitous computing with embedded virtuality, in Weiser's words:

> comes not from any one of these devices; it emerges from the interaction of all of them. The hundreds of processors and displays are not a user interface . . . [but] . . . a pleasant and effective 'place' to get things done . . . The technology required for ubiquitous computing comes in three parts: cheap, low-power computers that include equally convenient displays, a network that ties them all together, and software systems implementing ubiquitous applications . . . By pushing computers into the background, embodied virtuality will make individuals more aware of the people on the other ends of their computer links. This development carries the potential to reverse the unhealthy centripetal forces that conventional personal computers have introduced into life and the workplace.

Weiser looks forward to a world where computers are invisible, can promote calmness and can enhance connections between people, rather than the exact opposite.

Software developments

The Semantic Web

Sir Tim Berners-Lee, credited with inventing the world wide web by developing the hypertext program, has written about the 'Semantic Web'[3] within which:

> . . . for the Semantic Web to function, computers must have access to structured collections of information and sets of inference rules that they can use to conduct automated reasoning.

He continues . . .

> The real power of the Semantic Web will be realised when people create many programs that collect Web content from diverse sources, process the information and exchange the results with other programs. The effectiveness of such software agents will increase exponentially as

more machine-readable Web content and automated services (including other agents) become available.

Thus the change implied by this idea is that information on the World Wide Web which currently consists of documents for consumption by people will have to evolve to include data which can be processed automatically by machines. Berners-Lee foresees the Semantic Web extending into the physical world, and acting to enhance automation of all kinds, and ultimately extending human knowledge itself.

From this has sprung the idea of the Educational Semantic Web. Writing in the *Journal of Interactive Media in Education*,[4] the editors write about the three fundamental affordances on which it is based, the capacity for effective information storage and retrieval, the capacity for nonhuman autonomous 'agents' to augment the learning and information retrieval and processing power of human beings, and the capacity of the internet to support, extend and expand communications capabilities of humans in multiple formats across the bounds of time and space.

Adaptability, adaptivity and interactivity

Web-based resources will evolve to become more flexible for learners and to match learner characteristics. Systems will have to become both adaptive (the system includes flexible algorithms based on models of human behaviour to control content, presentation and navigation support) and adaptable by the user. A simple example of adaptivity from e-commerce is the 'Amazon' website which greets you by name and suggests purchases based on your own past purchasing behaviour. A simple example of adaptability is 'My Yahoo!', where any user who has logged on can personalise their own pages to influence both the appearance of the pages and their updated content, such as news bulletins.

Diana Laurillard, Professor of Educational Technology at the Open University, has formulated a set of requirements for educational media so that they can enhance the learning process.[5]

They should be:

- Discursive:
  - teacher's and students' conceptions are each accessible to the other and the topic goal is negotiable
  - students must be able to generate and receive feedback on descriptions appropriate to the topic goal
  - the teacher must be able to reflect on student's descriptions and adjust their own descriptions to be more meaningful to the student.
- Adaptive:
  - the teacher can use the relationship between their own and the student's conception to set up and adapt a task environment for the continuing dialogue, in the light of the topic goals
  - the student must be able to use their existing conceptual knowledge to adapt their actions in the task environment in order to achieve the task goal.
- Interactive:
  - the students can act within the task environment to achieve the task goal

– they should receive meaningful intrinsic feedback on their actions that relate to the nature of the task goal
– something in the environment must change in a meaningful way as a result of their actions.

- **Reflective:**
  – teachers must support the process by which students link the feedback on their actions to the topic goal i.e. link experience to descriptions of experience
  – the pace of the learning process must be controllable by the students, so that they can take the time needed to reflect on the task goal–action–feedback cycle in order to develop their conception in relation to the topic goal.

The language in this set of requirements is tailored to students in a higher education environment, but if the word 'system' is used for 'teacher', and the word 'learner' is used for 'student' then as a set of standards it is applicable to any e-learning environment. It is a theoretical standard which would be nearly impossible to realise fully in practical terms, but nonetheless is worthy of aspiration.

In the iClass project (www.iclass.info/iclass01.asp), the 'Intelligent distributed cognitive-based open learning system for schools' funded across the European Union, a hypermedia learning environment is being developed using a distillation of different models of learning styles, in order to create:

> An advanced learning system, founded on an ontology-based architecture for sequencing of knowledge, and adaptive to learner's level of understanding and learning style by dynamically creating individualized learning objects; [and] a distributed, collaborative environment with ubiquitous access for all . . . to rich multimedia content and services, empowering direct communication.

In this kind of system development interaction moves far beyond a simple question and answer format so that learners can begin to create their own learning environments in an interaction with systems, and our present Virtual Learning Environments (VLEs) will evolve into Personalised Learning Environments (PLEs).

At the School of Computer Science and Information Systems, Birkbeck College, London, Magoulas and colleagues are working on the development of educational hypermedia systems for the web, based on a 'synergy of computer science and instructional science', using individual differences between learners 'as a basis of system's adaptation'. They have moved from using learning styles to the concept of 'cognitive styles', as developed by Riding and Rayner[6] and others, and are now using:

> soft computing techniques [including] fuzzy logic, neural networks, genetic algorithms, fuzzy clustering and neuro-fuzzy systems . . . to handle and process human uncertainty and to simulate human decision-making.[7]

Trail records and navigational learning

What effect will the ideas and developments discussed above have on the future of e-learning? Peterson and Levene[8] describe the thinking behind the idea of 'trail records and navigational learning' as follows:

> Imagine again that you are a solicitor and that you are asked to provide internal advice to your firm on contract law in medicine. This is part of your lifelong learning: you studied aspects of contract law several years ago, and you now need to link this knowledge with new statutes and decisions concerning the medical sector. One of your colleagues has some knowledge of these links and provides useful pointers and references. After two weeks of work, you edit your materials together and construct a presentation for your firm. Two years later you are asked to revisit the same task including relevant updates and refinements.
>
> Imagine again that you are a tourist visiting a new city and its historic sites. Before the visit you use literature, maps and websites to prepare yourself. During the visit, you navigate around its sites, collecting a miscellany of notes, diaries, photographs and memories. When you return home you may try to edit these into some sort of ordered record. This record may be useful if you wish to remind yourself of what you did and saw, share your experiences with others, or prepare to revisit the same city. And it may contain links to other records, for example from a museum visit which you made long ago when you were at school.
>
> These examples of learning in different contexts show some interesting common features.
>
> 1 They all involve trails of learning objects. That is: the museum exhibits, the legal statutes, the tourist locations, and so on, are not encountered in isolation, but as elements in longer paths.
> 2 Some of the time we are engaged in enacting these trails: as we pass through the museum, undertake our course in contract law, or visit another site. We may be following a prescribed path from learning object to learning object, we may be creating something new and exploratory, or we may be doing a bit of both, but in any case we are 'on the ground' engaging in a series of experiences.
> 3 Some of the time we are engaged in editing our trails: as we plan them beforehand and refine and extend them afterwards, reflecting, reorganising and making and deleting connections. Thus, information becomes personal knowledge through a process of construction, and this process involves a cycle in which we enact, edit, re-enact and re-edit our trails.
>
> We will call this cycle 'navigational learning', using the general formulation: navigational learning = enactment + editing of trails'.

In our journey into the 'ambient' phase of computing, where computers are predicted to become a less visible and ever-present element of the environment, through the ubiquitous hardware described by Weiser, the semantic software of Berners-Lee, with 'intelligent agents' working 'to collect and transmit information, which work without our supervision, and which communicate and collaborate with each other', and the 'synergy of computer science and instructional science' being utilised by Magoulas and colleagues to create Personalised Learning Environments, then the potential of the computer to support learning is vastly extended.

Conclusion

A lot of what I have outlined in this chapter is currently in the realm of science fiction, but some of it will become fact and will change the way we live and work. None of the developers of interactive systems, however, expects computer-based Personalised Learning Environments to push other ways of learning to one side, and a general hope is expressed in the documentation for the work I have mentioned above that people will come together more and not less because of it. Let us hope that it can be so, as many of us feel a need to be encouraged that it is possible to see beyond the handicapping of interpersonal communication that our primary care clinical systems driven by government imperatives can so powerfully represent.

References

1 Hawisher GE (1992) Electronic meetings of the minds: research, electronic conferences, and composition studies. In: GE Hawisher and P LeBlanc (eds). *Re-imagining Computers and Composition: teaching and research in the virtual age*. Boynton/Cook, Portsmouth, New Hampshire.
2 Weiser M (1991) The computer for the 21st Century. *Scientific American*: 94–10, September. Available at: www.ubiq.com/hypertext/weiser/SciAmDraft3.html [last accessed 26 October 2005].
3 Berners-Lee T (2001) The Semantic Web – a new form of Web content that is meaningful to computers will unleash a revolution of new possibilities. *Scientific American*, pp. 34–43, May. Available at: www.ryerson.ca/~dgrimsha/courses/ cps720_02/resources/Scientific %20American%20The%20Semantic%20Web.htm [last accessed 26 October 2005].
4 Anderson T and Whitelock D (2004) The Educational Semantic Web: visioning and practising the future of education. *Journal of Interactive Media in Education*. 2004(1) (Special Issue on the Educational Semantic Web). Available at: www-jime.open.ac.uk/ 2004/1 [last accessed 26 October 2005].
5 Laurillard D (2002) *Rethinking University Teaching – a conversational framework for the effective use of learning technologies* (2e). RoutledgeFalmer, London.
6 Riding R and Rayner S (1998) *Cognitive Styles and learning Strategies*. David Fulton, London.
7 Frias-Martinez E, Magoulas G, Chen S and Macredie R (2005) Modelling Human Behaviour in User-Adaptive Systems: recent advances using soft computing techniques. *Expert Systems with Applications*. 29(2): 320–29. Available at: www.dcs.bbk.ac.uk/ ~gmagoulas/Modeling%20human%20behavior.pdf [last accessed 26 October 2005]. See also: www.dcs.bbk.ac.uk/~gmagoulas/publications.html.
8 Peterson DM and Levene M (2003) Trail records and navigational learning. *London Review of Education*. 1(3). Available at: www.dcs.bbk.ac.uk/selene/reports/trail_records_ and_navigational_learning.pdf [last accessed 26 October 2005].

Chapter 20

The opportunities and barriers to e-learning in education for primary care: a European perspective

Jochen Gensichen, Horst Christian Vollmar, Andreas C Soennichsen and Uta-Maria Waldmann

---

Key points

- The context of general practice and GP training in Germany offers exciting opportunities for e-learning.
- There is a wide variety in the quality of available e-learning approaches.
- Implementation is limited by lack of competence and confidence in both learners and educators.
- Poor co-ordination of e-learning development and financial sustainability lead to additional problems.

In the 1990s, the German government allocated millions of Euros for a variety of e-learning projects, including 13 major projects for e-learning in medical education. The hope was that it would produce significant benefits to both learners and educators.[1] We are now concerned that at the end of this governmental funding most of these promising projects will be dropped without having had the chance to demonstrate a sustainable effect on quality in medical education.

Potential benefits for primary care in Germany

There are some benefits of an e-learning approach to educational provision. One of the most useful benefits for e-learning in the general practice setting is that it can be delivered at any time and at any place. Also, it can be easily tailored to individual learning needs.[2–7] Since undergraduate and postgraduate education in general practice is organised as a community-based training it might particularly benefit from the flexibility of the e-learning approach.[8] Furthermore, the availability of e-learning in regions at large distance from university centres may help to motivate general practitioners (GPs) in rural areas to participate in continuing medical education (CME).[9]

GP training in Germany

University training (undergraduate)

The university curriculum comprises a six-year lecture-based programme. The first two years focus on the basic (medical) sciences and are followed by three years of lectures, courses and internships in the various medical subspecialties. In the last year of undergraduate medical education, the student spends the entire period in a clinical setting with three rotations in surgery, (internal) medicine and a specialty selected by the student. So far, general practice or primary care plays only a minor role in undergraduate medical education. Primary care departments are generally small and some universities do not have a department. All students have to complete one class of lectures and/or seminars in primary care and in most of the universities they have to attend only one mandatory one-week placement in a GP practice. Politicians have recognised the importance of strengthening general practice in medical education but the medical schools are very slow in turning the politically desired changes into reality.

The use of e-learning in undergraduate medical education is not generally well established. Electronic data processing is increasingly used for student administration as well as the planning and timing of classes and courses, but only a few faculties have implemented a thorough Learning Management System (LMS). Whenever e-learning approaches are used, they are used in an unsystematic way. Some lecturers do use the internet to offer additional information, such as by the use of PowerPoint presentations or PDF files, but e-learning is rarely integrated into the curriculum. Hardly any e-learning programmes with primary care specific content are in German and departments would need to create their own content, a time-consuming task. This could be facilitated by sharing of content with other departments, but would require a primary care specific solution for a group of universities or even on a national level. This rises the issues of the choice of a common programme as well as collaboration regarding funding, maintenance and support – barriers too high to be taken yet.

Vocational training (postgraduate)

After graduation from medical school the vocational training to become a GP comprises a five-year curriculum of training on the job in a clinical setting. The trainee spends three to four years working in the hospital (mainly in internal medicine, some time in surgery and electives). A period of community-based training for 18 months is provided in the practice of an experienced GP who acts as a trainer and supervisor. At present the clinical training of a GP-trainee is not structured. There are few vocational training schemes and most trainees have to organise their own rotations with positions as senior house officers in internal medicine, surgery and electives, as well as GP registrar posts. The learning content of the training varies widely from hospital to hospital as well as from practice to practice. Training is accompanied by an 80-hour curriculum organised by the German Medical Association, but its structure varies widely between the federal states. Protected teaching time or half-day release courses are rare. At the end of the training the general practice registrar has to pass an oral assessment, also administered by the Regional Medical Association.

In spite of its enormous potential, e-learning approaches are rarely applied in this setting. Trainees are spread all over the country and, especially in remote areas, they do not have access to academic medical facilities. An e-learning approach could definitely be useful in these circumstances, such as discussion boards, chat rooms or wikis, to improve professional communication.

Continuing medical education

In Germany working in general practice is characterised by some specific conditions: surgeries are mainly single-handed, although the number of group practices is increasing; GPs are self-employed with no capitation fee for registered patients; patients are free to choose and change their doctor at any time; it is difficult to work part-time or reduced hours to pursue other interests like teaching or special clinics; and a GP generally has to guarantee full-time availability for his patients. The possibility of job-sharing exists but it is associated with a drastic limitation of income. In January 2004 German health authorities introduced a structured approach to CME which requires that a certain amount of CME credits must be achieved within five years. If not, the GP faces a reduction in reimbursement or even the loss of the licence to practice. As a result of these events, web-based access to high quality medical education has become interesting for clinical practitioners.[10–13] This has prompted a variety of CME providers to launch web-based CME modules. Most of these are provided by medical journals that use their own published material, but there are also numerous offers of web-based CME that are sponsored by pharmaceutical companies. These e-learning units may be educationally effective but the content is mostly related to specific products.

Use and attitudes of primary care educators to e-learning

Our experience suggests that benefits will only be achieved if several important aspects are carefully considered. Many primary care educators are enthusiastic about e-learning but this is tempered by a variety of concerns. We recently investigated the use and attitudes of primary care educators to e-learning in Germany. The first national meeting on e-learning in general practice by the German Society of General Practice and Family Medicine was held in July 2005 and was followed by a survey using a Delphi technique.[14] The respondents were active in undergraduate and postgraduate education in primary care and can be considered innovators and early adaptors who are representative of those with high enthusiasm and commitment for e-learning.

Quality of e-learning products

There was an overall concern about the lack of assessment of educational quality or peer review of e-learning materials. There are international standards for technical aspects, but regarding the quality of its content and educational usefulness most e-learning materials have to be taken on trust by learners and educators alike. Often it is impossible to sufficiently preview them online to judge the quality since they may have specific access requirements. Very few e-learning products have been evaluated for their educational impact. It is difficult for educators and institutional providers to positively recommend e-learning materials in such circumstances.

Implementation of e-learning and attitudes of educators and learners

A common interest is how to integrate the various approaches of e-learning into existing educational provision and curricula. However, its implementation is restricted due to the lack of confidence and competence of both educators and learners in using these new techniques. Some educators appear to deny the inevitable spread of e-learning approaches into all aspects of education, including undergraduate medical education, and general practitioners mentioned fears that e-learning might replace clinical experiences of medical students with real-life patients in the future. This problem is made worse by the corresponding low levels of confidence and competence of both technology use and the e-learning approach in learners.

Curricula and lack of co-ordination

e-learning approaches have proliferated and are offered by a range of organisations. This may increase choice but it often results in a lack of sharing and co-ordination between the various providers. There may be several e-learning products that cover identical aspects of the same topic yet other topics are left with no provision. This is especially important when education for primary care is attempting to cover a curriculum that is prescribed by various institutions and professional organisations.

Time commitment

Another barrier mentioned by German educators is that the use and development of e-learning approaches is very time-consuming. Institutions and employers do not want to recognise that the development and implementation of e-learning modules takes at least as much time as the preparation of a traditional lecture. Learners also need time to become familiar and work with the e-leaning modules. Furthermore, e-learning has its own organisational prerequisites just like traditional learning approaches.

Funding and sustainability

A major concern is the level of funding for e-learning. Most e-learning approaches require an initial high level of resource allocation for development before subsequent economies can be realised. The concern is not only related to this initial funding but also to missing concepts of long-term funding for sustainability. Unfortunately most e-learning funding is associated with short-term development of projects and after completion of a project there are no funds and no concept of how to keep it up to date, to further improve it, and to implement it as a standard part of the curriculum.

The future of e-learning in German primary healthcare

Based on our experiences several key aspects will need to be considered if e-learning is to achieve its potential for primary care education in Germany. Quality standards for the educational aspects need to be developed, especially regarding user orientation and how the underlying educational approach has been used to enhance the content. e-learning material needs to be evaluated from the perspective of the learner and the educator. Integrating e-learning at an early stage of medical education could make it a natural part of a GP's lifelong learning, leading them from a more structured undergraduate curriculum to a self-directed postgraduate professional development.

However, e-learning is not a universal approach for medical education. It can never replace training in the real clinical setting, but it can offer a valuable method to enhance the learning experience, especially when a so-called blended learning approach is used.[15–19] Lessons learned require rapid publication to ensure that the findings influence educational policy and practice. GP educators wish to work more closely together and have organised themselves (German Network for e-Learning in General Practice). Barriers for content based e-learning programmes are not overcome yet, but sharing more flexible concepts is on the way.

e-learning: from hype into reality

One decade of German e-learning experiences shows various barriers and chances of the new technology in medical education. Now it is the time to turn the work from the hype of pilots to a systematic integration into the general practice training. For the next generation of general practitioners it should be the reality.

References

1 Fischer M (2003) E-learning in medical education, graduate and continuing medical education. Status and prospects [German]. *Medinische Klinik*. **98**(10): 594–7.
2 Schultze-Mosgau S, Zielinski T and Lochner J (2004) Web-based, virtual course units as a didactic concept for medical teaching. *Medical Teacher*. **26**(4): 336–42.
3 Clark D (2002) Psychological myths in e-learning. *Medical Teacher*. **24**(6): 598–604.
4 Asselmeyer H (2004) Trends, current developments, and concepts in distance learning and E-learning. *International Journal of Computers in Dentistry*. **7**(2): 145–57.
5 Davies D (2005) E-learning. In: J Dent and M Harden (eds). *A Practical Guide for Medical Teachers* (2e). Elsevier, Edinburgh.
6 Chumley-Jones H, Dobbie A and Alford C (2002) Web-based learning: sound educational method or hype? A review of the evaluation literature. *Academic Medicine*. **77**(10 Suppl): S86–93.
7 Cook D, Dupras D, Thompson W *et al.* (2005) Web-based learning in residents' continuity clinics: a randomized, controlled trial. *Academic Medicine*. **80**(1): 90–7.
8 Sandars J (2003) E-learning: the coming of age. *Education for Primary Care*. **14**: 1–5.
9 Butzlaff M, Vollmar HC, Floer B *et al.* (2004) Learning with computerized guidelines in general practice? A randomized controlled trial. *Family Practice*. **21**(2): 183–8.
10 Fordis M, King J, Ballantyne C *et al.* (2005) Comparison of the instructional efficacy of Internet-based CME with live interactive CME workshops: a randomized controlled trial. *Journal of the American Medical Association*. **294**(9): 1043–51.

11 Wiecha J and Barrie N (2002) Collaborative online learning: a new approach to distance CME. *Academic Medicine.* **5**: 756–7.

12 Mamary E and Charles P (2000) On-site to on-line: barriers to the use of computers for continuing education. *Journal of Continuing Education for Health Professionals.* **20**(3): 171–5.

13 Butzlaff M, Koneczny N, Floer B *et al.* (2002) Primary care physicians, internet and new knowledge. Utilization and efficiency of new educational media [German]. *Medizinische Klinik.* **97**(7): 383–8.

14 Schmidt UM, Sönnichsen A, Vollmar HC *et al.* (2005) *E-Learning in General Practice: barriers and chances in undergraduate and postgraduate medical training in Germany.* Proceedings of the AMEE 2005, Amsterdam NL.

15 Cook D (2005) The research we still are not doing: an agenda for the study of computer-based learning. *Academic Medicine.* **80**(6): 541–8.

16 Gold JP, Begg WB, Fullerton D *et al.* (2004) Successful implementation of a novel internet hybrid surgery curriculum: the early phase outcome of thoracic surgery prerequisite curriculum e-learning project. *Annals of Surgery.* **240**(3): 499–507.

17 Shaffer K and Small J (2004) Blended learning in medical education: use of an integrated approach with web-based small group modules and didactic instruction for teaching radiologic anatomy. *Academic Radiology.* **11**(9): 1059–70.

18 Gordon D, Issenberg S, Gordon M *et al.* (2005) Stroke training of prehospital providers: an example of simulation-enhanced blended learning and evaluation. *Medical Teacher.* **27**(2): 114–21.

19 Karnath B, Das Carlo M and Holden M (2004) A comparison of faculty-led small group learning in combination with computer-based instruction versus computer-based instruction alone on identifying simulated pulmonary sounds. *Teaching in Learning and Medicine.* **16**(1): 23–7.

Chapter 21

Educational research and e-learning: responding to the challenge

Jonathan Burton and Anne McKee

Key points

- Little original research about e-learning in primary care has been published.
- The aim of research is to stimulate debate and of promote better practice.
- The approaches to research on e-learning are no different from any other piece of educational research.
- Publication of findings from research can influence wider policies and procedures.

Introduction

A useful definition of research is that it is involves the systematic investigation of the subject under study. Often, the researcher, in undertaking the investigation, aims to both learn more about the subject and evaluate aspects of it. The words 'systematic', 'investigation' and 'evaluation' indicate a degree of orderliness, thoroughness and critique that frame an enquiry. These descriptors emphasise that the work has followed a carefully thought out design, approach to collecting evidence, analysis and reporting.

In the real world, all researchers have to undertake research within the constraints of what is possible in practice. This has an impact upon the scope of the enquiry – what can reasonably be investigated, learnt and claimed. Even when the scope and intention of an enquiry is carefully planned, unanticipated events and challenges will be encountered. It is the unexpected which often necessitates changes to initial intentions and schedules. Making clear what challenges were encountered, and why plans had to be changed helps to keep the orderliness and thoroughness of the enquiry. This applies equally to small- and large-scale research because both encounter the unexpected.

Different kinds of research can be valued differently. This should not be confused with one kind of research being better than another. Qualitative research is becoming more accepted in medical education but it is often not trusted or understood as much as quantitative approaches. The science of medicine is based upon quantitative forms of research. Trained within the discipline of medicine, doctors often have higher levels of confidence in this kind of research, they value it more. The growing popularity of qualitative research reflects an opening of minds to a different perspective and its contribution. Perhaps, more critical than the difference in how quantitative and qualitative research is valued is the difference between large-scale 'expert' research and practitioner research. The former is often regarded as 'proper, valid research', the latter as amateur dabbling around practice from which the practitioner might learn something. As we have suggested earlier in this chapter, the principles of systematic enquiry apply to both. Practitioner research can be quantitative or qualitative or pursue mixed methodological approaches. It is often smaller in scale, and more keenly focused upon application to practice. In the journal *Work Based Learning in Primary Care*, we have endeavoured to encourage the publication of practitioner research because it articulates what professionals learn through practice and the investigation of practice. Guidelines to authors imply a basic and general approach to systematic enquiry.

Box 21.1 Instructions for contributors to the 'Practitioner Research Section': *Work Based Learning in Primary Care*

Practitioner research should be about the practitioner's own involvement in learning or developing practice in the work setting. Pieces of work by new researchers are welcome. Conclusions from the study might cover such areas as lessons for future learning and points for patient care.

There is an established literature on practitioner research (sometimes called action research) in schooling and an evolving one in health sciences.[1–4] The utility of practitioner research is that it enables professional development, supports a considered approach to changing practice and has the capacity to identify and enhance practice-based learning.

The usefulness of original published writing is a quality which is emphasised by John Pitts in writing about the journal which he edits (*Education in Primary Care*). He says, 'feedback about this journal is couched in terms of usefulness, relevance and practicality.'[5] He wonders what sort of papers are going to be read by his audience. He believes that they have to be useful to the journal's audience and he gives a list of the criteria by which educational research may be judged for a journal such as his (*see* Box 21.2).

Box 21.2 Attributes for judging educational research – adapted from John Pitts[5]

1   About education in the broadest sense.
2   Practical/of use/intelligible and informative to others.
3   Should help both professional development and the growth of knowledge about education (in both the author-researcher and the reader).
4   Transferable or of use to similar situations.
5   Contribute to the reinforcement of existing knowledge.

A journal such as *Education for Primary Care* or *Work Based Learning in Primary Care* has to make sure that its contents are practical and of use to its audience. This does not mean to say that the journals should not stretch their readership. They should. But journals such as these are largely about practical aspects of learning and education in primary care, as seen by those who are concerned about and involved in the issues they write about.

Research into learning

If you are researching into the learning of others, you are dealing with something which is slippery to define and capture. It is also subject to a large number of variables. Research into learning is research into one aspect of human behaviour, which is subject to a range of influences at one point in time, and a larger range of influences over a lifetime. A particular educational input, such as a day course, may not be the only influence on the subsequent behaviour of the participating learner. The learner may also be reading journals and other professional literature in their own time. The learner may be discussing their work with colleagues. Cultural and personal issues will also influence the individual learner. These factors may augment and deepen the knowledge and skills gained from the day course, without being in any way a part of that course. Equally these factors may have a negative impact on what is learned and how that knowledge is used. In summary, there can be a number of influences on people's learning behaviour and for this reason it cannot always be true that an educational input will lead to a foreseeable result or a result that can be causally linked to the input. Equally, the fact that your sample population has 'learned' something does not necessarily mean that they will be able to use that in their actual practice or retain it over time. Bear these ideas in mind before you too readily link particular outcomes to particular input. Learning does not take place in controlled laboratory settings nor can it be controlled or predicted. At best it can be facilitated and enabled.

e-learning in general practice

There is an enormous amount of e-learning going on inside and outside general practice, both formally and informally. Is this changing how we can and are learning? Is it changing our expectations of how we should best learn?

An informal survey of GP appraisers, presented by Professor Peter Orton at the Royal College of General Practitioners conference 'Developing the future of e-learning in primary care: responding to the challenge' (15 March 2005), found that e-learning contributes to 70% of continuing professional development (CPD) for this group. This unpublished research suggests that e-learning is the most commonly used form of learning for the Professional Development Plans (PDPs) of GPs and that other forms of learning such as chalk and talk sessions in postgraduate centres and even practice-based learning meetings are on the wane.

There are many different modes of e-learning. Each of these constitutes an important learning strategy, potentially to be used by GPs:

- self-directed learning using search engines such as Google or other forms of web-quests
- CD-ROM

- computer-based learning, which may be moderated or non-moderated
- collaborative learning – either synchronous or asynchronous
- blended e-learning – where e-learning is combined with another form of learning – for example, attending a course
- communities of practice and learning networks, which could be created or natural
- the use of simulated learning environments.

It is appropriate to ask whether the current approaches to e-learning in primary care make the most of the capacity of the technology. There are two aspects to this question. One is about the optimal use of the technology. Are people using it well and with ease? Does it meet their needs and preferences? The other aspect is about whether the technology is enabling people to do things differently or to do different things. How does e-learning effect how people learn and interact with others in virtual environments?

In *Is there anybody there? The embodiment of knowledge in virtual environments* Rob Walker has asked if e-learning is innovation without change.[6] By that he meant, have the conventions and approaches of traditional teaching have been transformed in e-learning or not? It is an important question because a lot is known about the strengths and limitations of traditional teaching practice and its resistance to change. Are those interested in education and learning dealing with something akin to what they already know about learning and teaching, or is e-learning a different phenomenon?

Rob Walker asks:

- Has the computer replaced or displaced the teacher?
- Does the web page replace or displace the book?
- Does the e-conference replace or displace the seminar and classroom?
- Does email replace or displace the tutorial?

Rob emphasises the potential of technology to recast the roles of teacher and learner and make teaching and learning processes transparent. He argues persuasively that there is potential for significant pedagogic change. But how much of this potential is realised? In the early stages of innovation, what is new is often understood by reference to what has been. Rob tries to allude to the change in e-learning by questioning how it is different from or the same as traditional teaching and learning. These questions push us towards identifying what is different and unique about the e-learning process and how people do and might engage with it. It is important to ask these kinds of questions because investigating them will help us to understand how best to design and use e-learning.

Two key advantages of e-learning are its accessibility and up-to-dateness. e-learning can be undertaken anytime, anywhere and this may be a major reason for the growing popularity of e-learning amongst GPs. With regards to content, there is, potentially, less risk of information becoming obsolescent, as internet-based educational content can be easily changed.

There are barriers to e-learning. Computers and software are essential and, for some, these are not easily accessible or affordable. Users may be unfamiliar with the software either because they are novice or because updated software has new features compromised by teething problems. Other problems include learners' lack of confidence/competence, and the difficulty for some learners to access a computer and achieve what is called connectivity.

An example of research into e-learning

So far in this chapter, we have described some of the key issues in research and, in particular, into research into learning. We have described some aspects of the world of e-learning. We are now going to help the reader with a practical example of research into e-learning and hopefully demonstrate some of the themes we have already raised.

Box 21.3 Example of a research project: 'Evaluating the doctors.net.uk model of electronic continuing medical education'[7]

Doctors.net.uk and bmjlearning.com are providers of internet-based, non-moderated learning. The format of the most commonly provided modules is remarkably similar between each of these providers, with a format based on some instruction and with assessment by before and after knowledge testing via MCQ or similar. This format builds on traditional modes of medical education that concentrate upon providing information and testing recall and comprehension. With doctors.net.uk, a pass mark of 70% qualifies the participant for a certificate of completion. These providers are both widely used by general practitioners. For example, between April 2003 and March 2004, 7548 unique GPs successfully completed e-learning modules offered by doctors.net.uk. In this paper, the authors wished to describe and analyse the learning engendered by the modules of doctors.net.uk. They show how in two e-learning modules on the subject of irritable bowel syndrome, taken between 2001 and 2004 by 3070 doctors, the participants have improved their scores in the before and after knowledge assessments from 68.4% to 86.7% in the first module and from 73% to 79% in the second module. But as the authors rightly state, the improved scores reported in their paper are not evidence of improved outcomes for patients. Indeed, they allude to the fact that the short-term retention of knowledge (measured by the before and after assessments) may not even indicate any long-term change to the basis of the participants' knowledge.

Sue Lacey Bryant and Tim Ringrose's paper does demonstrate many of the themes that have already been discussed.[7] First, the authors are enthusiastic about a learning medium, in which they have been professionally involved and which has been widely used by GPs. Their data shows that participants have improved their short-term knowledge. However, the authors are sensible not to make too many claims as to how effective these modules are, beyond the fact that participants' short-term knowledge is improved. The modules may indeed be very effective but doctors.net.uk simply does not know whether the new short-term knowledge has been sustained in the long term, nor do they know whether patient care has been improved at all. The quality of their research writing does depend on their capacity to raise these critical questions. And, for the reader who is interested in e-learning, the most important lesson from this paper may come from the brief discussion at the end of the paper. In this, the authors put forward some ideas as to how the sort of e-learning promoted by doctors.net.uk might be transmuted into such desirable long-term outcomes, such as improving patient care.

Thinking about becoming an author: advice for novice and not so novice authors

Research is often generated and inspired by enthusiasm. This enthusiasm may be sparked by a perfectly laudable ambition to 'showcase' what can be or has been achieved in a particular field of activity or the advantages of one way of doing things. We are all enthusiasts in our lives and this helps motivate us to contribute and share, which is fundamental to research.

Many of you who are working in general practice as practitioners and educators may feel unsure at the thought of writing for a research journal. Your enthusiasm may be tempered by doubt.

It is, indeed, a challenging task, for your expertise in clinical and managerial matters has not necessarily prepared you for the task of journal writing. It is not an easy task to write, in say 2500 words, a succinct and appropriately referenced piece of work.

But let us look at your advantages. You may well be working at the coal face, in that ever unfolding drama which is general practice, Your working life is replete with practical and very interesting experiences from which you are learning. You are used to thinking systematically: for example, you are used to doing audit. If you are a GP you will know the difference between the construction of a well thought out referral letter about a patient and one which is a little sloppy. A good letter communicates clearly, succinctly and accurately, and you will feel proud about the effort you have put into it. A sloppy letter is a bit of a muddle, and when you re-read it you find that it is unclear and that you may have left out important information. Some of you will have written a dissertation for a Master's degree, some of you will have written up a project as GP registrars. So you have a rich world ripe for practice-based research, and to an extent you will have had experience in constructing a good piece of writing. Now you may wish to go one step further by writing a paper for a peer-reviewed journal. You will want that writing to disseminate your learning, and to articulate it in ways that will be more considered and analytical than the types of writing referred to earlier in this paragraph.

It is worth looking positively at your advantages. Compare yourself with a non-medical, research educationalist. A research educationalist does not have the rich world of general practice immediately at hand, and has to go out to do field work in other people's daily work places. You have the advantage of immediacy and of being an insider. This is your world and you know things about it that take time and participation in that world to get to know. Outside researchers will report impartially on a world they observe and, usually, will leave. You live in that world, are affected by what happens in it. That will include reactions to your research and any changes it may help stimulate.

Many journals now encourage a less formal style of writing than what we will call traditional formal academic writing. Formal academic writing has been replete with the passive tense, uneasy with the use of the first person and often framed in specialised language that seems remote from ordinary everyday English. We would encourage you to write, 'I started this study because I was interested in . . .' rather than 'This study seeks to investigate . . .'. In most journals which publish papers on education you can abandon the IMRAD structure (Introduction, Methods, Results and Discussion) if that feels better for you. Choose a structure that enables you to say what you feel needs to be said. The key task is not to say all that can be said but to say what most needs to be said about your study. Many journals have significant non-peer-reviewed sections and this might be a place to begin writing for. But there is one important thought to carry through: all writing is about communicating clearly and succinctly with the reader, whether it is the referral letter, or the sweated over first paper which you submit to a peer-reviewed journal.

We have just mentioned the dreaded words 'peer review'. The editors of many journals will look at your paper informally, and give you advice, before you submit for peer review. If you formally submit your research paper to a journal, it is first read by one of a core editorial team, who will then ask two of their peer reviewers to review the paper. To pass the process of peer review should be seen as a triumph – but a triumph that is likely to take some time. Peer reviewers require that almost all authors amend their papers. So if you sail through without being asked to rewrite to an extent, you have done something unusual. Do not feel bad about being asked to amend your paper. Peer reviewers are often chosen because they know a lot about the area you are writing about. Their feedback begins the process of you making your learning public and they are there to help by shaping your paper to be the best it can. Some e-journals recognise that the peer review process contributes to understanding and debate on a subject by putting the exchanges between peer-reviewers and authors online.[8] This is one example of how e-publishing might transform how research is reported. Peer review begins a conversation about a paper, rather than confine itself to a compromise between author and reviewer about what needs to be said and how.

Before you submit your paper, think carefully about the chances of it being selected. If you submit to the *British Medical Journal* your chances of being accepted are very low, perhaps 7%, whereas if you submit to *Education for Primary Care* or *Work Based Learning in Primary Care*, your chances of eventually being published are somewhat over 70%. Other journals lie in between. Think also about who would be interested in your paper and this can help you prioritise which journals to send your paper too.

Journals like *Education for Primary Care* or *Work Based Learning in Primary Care* also specialise in publishing papers by professionals who are also educators and their readership tends to come from the same background. Knowing what kind of audience the journal you choose serves will help you choose a writing style.

What type of papers will be considered for publication in a peer-reviewed journal on education or learning? Some, but not all, published papers will involve a degree of field research. Some journals encourage the publication of papers based on MSc dissertations. All the journals we have mentioned publish papers, which are ideas or discussion papers – these papers are referenced but have not involved any original field research. All these different approaches can be counted as research.

Conclusion

In this chapter, we have written generally about research and research into learning. We have looked particularly at practitioner research and have mentioned the other forms of research writing, which will be considered by peer-reviewed journals. We have explained that, in doing research, enthusiasm and resilience help. But we have suggested that good researchers need to stand aside from their enthusiasm and investment in their project. Failure to treat their results impartially or in a balanced way can lead to failing to persuade the reader that they have something worthwhile to share, that there is something worthwhile to learn from their work. A danger is that the potential learning from the project is limited because the more uncomfortable lessons or shortcomings are glossed over or ignored.

Writing a piece of research on an e-learning subject is no different from any other piece of educational research writing. The mode of learning may be different but the uncertainties are just the same. You have to ask yourself the same questions: have I made the setting and background of my study clear to the reader, what do my findings show, how can I comment on these, what sense can I make from what I have found out?

The written word is a powerful way of communicating with others, of stimulating debate and of promoting better practice. Research can ask important questions or suggest important information. Such questions and information should get into the public domain, where they can have the wider influence they deserve. Very little original research about e-learning in primary care has been published, although it is clear that e-learning is widely used. Hopefully this situation will change over the next few years.

References

1 Day C, Elliott J, Somekh B and Winter R (eds) (2002) *Theory & Practice in Action Research*. Symposium Books, Oxford.
2 Altrichter H, Posch P and Somekh B (1993) *Teachers Investigate Their Work*. Routledge, London.
3 McNiff J (1994) *Action Research: Principles and Practice*. Routledge, London.
4 Hart E and Bond M (1995) *Action Research for Health and Social Care*. Open University Press, Buckingham.
5 Pitts J (2004) 'Judging educational research' and the selection of papers for publication. *Education for Primary Care*. **15**: 143–9.
6 Walker R (2002) Is there anyone there? The embodiment of knowledge in virtual environments. Paper written for C Vrasidas and G Glass (eds) *Current Perspective on Applied Information Technologies, Vol 1 Distance Learning*. www.uea.ac.uk/care/people/RW-recnt-writings.
7 Lacey Bryant S and Ringrose T (2005). Evaluating the doctors.net.uk model of electronic continuing medical education. *Work Based Learning in Primary Care*. **3**: 129–42.
8 Summers T (2002) Promoting scholarship through design. In: WH Dutton and BD Loader (eds). *Digital Academe: the new media and higher education and learning*. Routledge, London.

Index

Page numbers in *italic* refer to figures.